THE ROCKEFELLER FOUNDATION, PUBLIC HEALTH AND INTERNATIONAL DIPLOMACY, 1920–1945

Studies for the Society for the Social History of Medicine

Series Editors: David Cantor
Keir Waddington

Titles in this Series

1 Meat, Medicine and Human Health in the Twentieth Century
David Cantor, Christian Bonah and Matthias Dörries (eds)

2 Locating Health: Historical and Anthropological Investigations of Place and Health
Erika Dyck and Christopher Fletcher (eds)

3 Medicine in the Remote and Rural North, 1800–2000
J. T. H. Connor and Stephan Curtis (eds)

4 A Modern History of the Stomach: Gastric Illness, Medicine and British Society, 1800–1950
Ian Miller

5 War and the Militarization of British Army Medicine, 1793–1830
Catherine Kelly

6 Nervous Disease in Late Eighteenth-Century Britain: The Reality of a Fashionable Disorder
Heather R. Beatty

7 Desperate Housewives, Neuroses and the Domestic Environment, 1945–1970
Ali Haggett

8 Disabled Children: Contested Caring, 1850–1979
Anne Borsay and Pamela Dale (eds)

9 Toxicants, Health and Regulation since 1945
Soraya Boudia and Nathalie Jas (eds)

10 A Medical History of Skin: Scratching the Surface
Jonathan Reinarz and Kevin Patrick Siena (eds)

11 The Care of Older People: England and Japan, A Comparative Study
Mayumi Hayashi

12 Child Guidance in Britain, 1918–1955: The Dangerous Age of Childhood
John Stewart

13 Modern German Midwifery, 1885–1960
Lynne Fallwell

14 Western Maternity and Medicine, 1880–1990
Janet Greenlees and Linda Bryder (eds)

15 Human Heredity in the Twentieth Century
Bernd Gausemeier, Staffan Müller-Wille and Edmund Ramsden (eds)

16 Biologics, A History of Agents Made From Living Organisms in the Twentieth Century
Alexander von Schwerin, Heiko Stoff and Bettina Wahrig (eds)

17 Bacteria in Britain, 1880–1939
Rosemary Wall

18 Health and Citizenship: Political Cultures of Health in Modern Europe
Frank Huisman and Harry Oosterhuis (eds)

19 The Politics of Hospital Provision in Early Twentieth-Century Britain
Barry M. Doyle

20 Institutionalizing the Insane in Nineteenth-Century England
Anna Shepherd

21 Psychiatry and Chinese History
Howard Chiang (ed.)

22 The Development of Scientific Marketing in the Twentieth Century: Research for Sales in the Pharmaceutical Industry
Jean-Paul Gaudillère and Ulrike Thoms (eds)

23 Stress in Post-War Britain, 1945–85
Mark Jackson (ed.)

Forthcoming Titles

The Politics of Vaccination: A Global History
Christine Holmberg, Stuart Blume and Paul R. Greenough (eds)

THE ROCKEFELLER FOUNDATION, PUBLIC HEALTH AND INTERNATIONAL DIPLOMACY, 1920–1945

BY

Josep L. Barona

Routledge
Taylor & Francis Group
LONDON AND NEW YORK

First published in paperback 2024

First published 2015 by Pickering & Chatto (Publishers) Limited

Published 2016 by Routledge
4 Park Square, Milton Park, Abingdon, Oxon OX14 4RN

and by Routledge
605 Third Avenue, New York, NY 10158

Routledge is an imprint of the Taylor & Francis Group, an informa business

BRITISH LIBRARY CATALOGUING IN PUBLICATION DATA

Barona Vilar, Josep Lluis, author.
Th e Rockefeller Foundation, public health and international diplomacy, 1920–1945. – (Studies for the Society for the Social History of Medicine)
1. Public health – Europe – History – 20th century. 2. Rockefeller Foundation
3. League of Nations
I. Title II. Series
362.1'094'09042-dc23

ISBN: 978-1-84893-567-9 (hbk)
ISBN: 978-1-03-292675-9 (pbk)
ISBN: 978-1-315-65367-9 (ebk)

DOI: 10.4324/9781315653679

Typeset by Pickering & Chatto (Publishers) Limited

CONTENTS

ACKNOWLEDGEMENTS

This book is the result of research conducted in the frame of two research projects: 'International Health and the Transfer of Scientific Knowledge: Europe 1900–75' [funded by the Spanish Government, MINECO, HAR2011–23233] and 'The Transfer of Scientific Knowledge on Health: Hunger, Nutrition and Vaccines, 1900–75' [funded by the Generalitat Valenciana, Prometeo 2012/056]. The main research work has been conducted at the League of Nations Library and Archives (Palais des Nations, Geneva) and at the Rockefeller Archive Centre (Sleepy Hollow, NY). I am particularly grateful to the Rockefeller Foundation, which contributed a Research Grant-in-Aid. I would like to thank Mark Pollard and Keir Waddington for editorial comments and Josep Bernabeu (Universitat d'Alacant), Ximo Guillem (Universitat de València), Astri Andresen (University of Bergen), Bartolomé Yun Casalillas (European University Institute, Florence) and Mark Harrison (University of Oxford) for bracing discussions and fruitful suggestions. The author is most grateful to Jacques Oberson (League of Nations Archives), Lee R. Hiltzik, Assistant Director and Head of Donor Relations and Collection Development (Rockefeller Archive Centre) as well as Bethany J. Antos (Archivist, Rockefeller Archive Centre), for their kind collaboration and help in the management of archival documents.

LIST OF TABLES

ABBREVIATIONS

HO: Health Organization
HC: Health Committee
HS: Health Section
IEIS: International Epidemiological Intelligence Service
IHA: International Health Agency
IHB: International Health Board
IHD: International Health Division
ILO: International Labour Office
LN: League of Nations
LNHO: League of Nations Health Organization
OIHP: Office Internationale d'Hygiène Publique
RF: Rockefeller Foundation
WHO: World Health Organization

A NOTE ON THE PRINCIPAL CHARACTERS

Avenol, Joseph Louis, was a French diplomat. He served as the second Secretary General of the League of Nations from 3 July 1933 to 31 August 1940. He was preceded by Eric Drummond of the United Kingdom, who was general secretary between 1920 and 1933. Avenol was sent to the League of Nations from the French Treasury Department in 1922 to handle the League's finances.

Bernard, Léon, was one of the founders of the Health Organization of the League of Nations as a delegate of the French Government. He actively participated in international public health initiatives, interchange of health officers and was the proponent of an international school of hygiene in Paris. Bernard pioneered nutrition as an essential field of public health during the great Depression.

Biraud, Yves, was a French expert for epidemiology acting as director of the International Epidemiological Intelligence Service of the League of Nations. He made contributions in the field of nutrition for public health.

Boudreau, Frank, was born of American parents in Quebec. He worked in the Ohio State Department of Health from 1911 to 1917, then served in the Army Medical Corps as a major and, in 1925, went to Geneva, eventually becoming the Director of the League of Nations Health Section.

Buchanan, George, was a senior Medical Officer at the British Ministry of Health and British delegate at the *Office Internationale d'Hygiène Publique*; he was appointed as Vice-President of the Health Committee of the League of Nations

Chodzko, Witold, was a Polish medical activist and psychiatrist. Appointed Minister of Heath in Poland (1919), closely linked to Ludwik Rajchman, he strengthened relations with the Health Organization of the League of Nations and actively participated in the creation of the National School of Hygiene in Warsaw.

Drummond, James Eric, was the first Secretary-General of the League of Nations. Drummond participated as a member of the British delegation to the Paris Peace Conference of 1919 and he was involved in the drafting of the Covenant of the League of Nations. With strong backing from British and American leaders, he was appointed League Secretary-General in May 1919.

Gautier, Raymond, was a Swiss public health expert and director of the University Institute of Hygiene and Bacteriology in Geneva. He joined the League of Nations in 1924, working on biological standardization. Between 1926 and 1930 he acted as director of the Far East Bureau in Singapore. In 1939 he became acting director of the Health Section and, from 1942 until the end of the war, he was entrusted with missions to London and Washington to rearrange public health in the liberated territories of Europe. When the World Health Organization Interim Commission became established in 1946, Gautier became first counsellor, a few months later he was appointed Director of the Geneva Office and in 1948 assumed the role of Assistant Director-General of the permanent Organization.

Gates, Frederick, was an American Baptist clergyman, and the principal business and philanthropic advisor to the major oil industrialist and philanthropist John D. Rockefeller from 1891 to 1923. He proved to be central to the suggestion and subsequent design of the funding plans for the creation, by Rockefeller, of the Baptist University of Chicago. Since 1912 Gates focused exclusively on philanthropy. In 1901 Gates designed the *Rockefeller Institute for Medical Research* (now Rockefeller University) of which he was board president, and then the Rockefeller Foundation, becoming a trustee upon its creation in 1913.

Grotjahn, Alfred, was a German physician becoming the first appointed chair of Social Hygiene at the Humboldt University of Berlin in 1920. Grotjahn was a Social Democrat leader of the 'anti-Nordic' wing of the German eugenics movement. He proposed and developed the concept of *Soziale Pathologie*.

Gunn, Selskar. Born in London, England, in 1883, Selskar Gunn led a distinguished career with the Rockefeller Foundation that involved him in some of the most important issues of his day. He became an American citizen in 1906 and subsequently held a number of positions in the field of public health before becoming an officer of the RF. In 1917 he was sent to France to act as Associate Director of the Commission for Prevention of Tuberculosis in France. In 1920 Gunn headed to Czechoslovakia to serve as an advisor to that nation's Public Health Administration. In 1922 the RF reassigned Gunn to the Paris office of the RF to assume the directorship of divisional operations for all of Europe. Gunn remained a member of the International Health Division until 1927.

Madsen, Thornvald, was a Danish physician and bacteriologist director of *Statens Serum Institut* (State Institute of Serum) from 1910 to 1940. During the Great War Madsen was heavily involved in humanitarian work for prisoners. From 1916 onwards Madsen did several inspection visits to detention centres in Russia. In the years 1921–37 Madsen was president of the League of Nations Health Committee.

Newman, George, was a public health expert, Quaker, the first Chief Medical Officer to the Ministry of Health in England and, as public health expert of the League of Nations, he was an active contributor to the creation of the Far East Bureau in Singapore.

Prausnitz, Carl. German physician, bacteriologist and hygienist. Prausnitz moved to London in 1905, and became an instructor at the Royal Institute of Public Health. He actively participated in the programs for the instruction of public health experts implemented by the RF and the HO.

Rajchman, Ludwik, a Jewish Polish bacteriologist, after graduating in Krakow, majored in microbiology at the Pasteur Institute (Paris). Between 1910 and 1913 Rajchman taught bacteriology at the Kings College (London). During the Great War he became the head of the Central Laboratory of dysentery (London). In 1918 he returned to Warsaw and founded the National Institute of Hygiene and the National School of Health (1923) funded by the Rockefeller Foundation. Rajchman was a great promoter of international health and was the director of the Organization of Hygiene for the League of Nations.

Rockefeller, John D. American billionaire, as the founder of the Standard Oil Company. Motivated by religious conviction, he used his fortune to establish several philanthropic institutions. In 1889 Frederick Gates asked for his help in establishing a great Baptist university, the University of Chicago. Gates worked as philanthropic advisor. In 1896 John D. Rockefeller retired from the active leadership of Standard Oil and devoted himself more entirely to philanthropy. Over the next decade, he and Gates created projects intended to cope with and solve social and medical problems. In 1901 The Rockefeller Institute for Medical Research was founded, followed by the General Education Board in 1902 and the Rockefeller Sanitary Commission in 1909. Seeking a more comprehensive approach to philanthropy, John D. Rockefeller created The Rockefeller Foundation in 1913 with an original endowment of $100 million.

Rose, Wickliffe, was a professor of history and philosophy at Peabody College and the University of Nashville. Rose's association with Rockefeller organizations began in 1910 with his appointment as Executive Secretary of the Rockefeller Sanitary Commission. As a result of his success with the RSC, Rose was appointed one of the original trustees of the Rockefeller Foundation in 1913. He also served as Chairman of the War Relief Commission during the Great War and General Director of the International Health Board from 1915 to 1923. Rose also helped to found public health schools at Johns Hopkins University and Harvard, and assisted in the founding the London School of Hygiene and Tropical Medicine.

Russell, Frederick, was directly responsible for introducing the typhoid vaccine to United States Army troops in 1910. When Rose stepped down as IHB director in 1923, Russell replaced him, promoting a more technological and laboratory approach to public health which emphasized the importance of scientific research to improve public health and served as the basis for successful disease control programs.

Stampar, Andreja, was the Director of the National School of Hygiene in Zagreb. He acted as public health officer at the Health Organization of the League of Nations and was a fellow of the Rockefeller Foundation. He also was involved in the League programs in China.

Strode, George K. Director of the Rockefeller Foundation's International Health Division in the Paris Office.

Sydenstriker, Edgar, worked in the United States Public Health Service, was the director of the International Intelligence Epidemiology Service of the League of Nations in Geneva and worked for the Milbank Memorial Fund. In the United States Public Health Service he worked on studies about pellagra until being appointed in 1920 chief of the Office of Statistical Investigations.

Theiler, Max, was a specialist in Tropical Medicine at the Harvard Medical School. In 1930 joined the staff of the IHD of the Rockefeller Foundation and developed a vaccine against yellow fever in 1936; he became Director of Laboratories of the Rockefeller Foundation's Division of Medicine and Public Health in 1951, the same year when he was awarded with the Nobel Prize for his research on yellow fever.

Vincent, George E., was second president of the Rockefeller Foundation (1917–29). As president he supported the continued expansion of the RF's public health activities, including the creation of the RF's Division of Medical Education, and oversaw a major reorganization of the Foundation into five divisions in 1928. In addition to his role as RF President and Trustee, Vincent was a member of the General Education Board, Peking Union Medical College and the China Medical Board.

White, Norman, was a Medical Officer serving at the League of Nations Health Section and an active participant in the creation of the International Epidemiological Intelligence Bureau for the as head of the Far East. He was the main coordinator of the Sanitary Convention for the Far East (1922). He also participated in the creation of a National School of Hygiene in Greece.

INTRODUCTION

The huge crisis caused by the Great War and the Interwar period radically changed the international relations affecting the social, economic and political situation in many European countries.[1] Health problems directly linked to the impairment of the living conditions and the loss of quality of life standards figured prominently as the authorities had to cope with the deep social crisis suffered by European countries during the first decades of the twentieth century. The challenge required a shift from the traditional public health control of plagues and infectious diseases to a more political issue represented by the development of social hygiene and social medicine.[2]

Several important features were involved in this shift: first, the role of international health organizations as a new locus of expertise. The international context determined the orientation of medical research and health policies anywhere in the world. In addition, international organizations played an important role in the standardization of research and clinical methods, and in the instructive programs for public health experts. These experts had an increasing influence on the organization of research in the several aspects involved in public health, health care and health policies at the national administrations and international agencies. Not only did experts and specialists acquire great scientific and political legitimacy and influence, health itself became a prominent social and political category during the pre-war years, during wartime and throughout the post-war period, a time when the State strongly emerged as a social regulator in most liberal societies in order to palliate the negative effects of the so called *market failures*.[3] The growing influence of the international networks and organizations on national health policies prompted the relevance of debates and negotiations in the shaping of preventing diseases and implementing health care strategies.

Some historians have considered the role of international agencies in the promotion of social medicine – for example, the Rockefeller Foundation (RF), the League of Nations Health Organization (LNHO), the Red Cross and a series of philanthropic and activist organizations in the field of health – as a strategy associated with Western imperialism, economic profit and political interests. A meaningful part of the historiography has considered American philanthropy as a key agent in the global spreading of capitalism and in the Western imperialist expansion.[4] It has been highlighted that the interests of colonial powers, big corporations and financial trusts took priority in international politics over those of native populations who were affected, assuming without any sort of criticism that both shared the same idea of development and that their respective interests were coincident. Indeed criticism is necessary to prevent the consideration that Western philanthropic foundations and their activists were working to advance good causes in a disinterested way. However, it has been recognized that most philanthropic institutions, and particularly the RF, helped to modernize world societies – promoting public health policies, improvements in agriculture, giving impulse to scientific research and instruction-grant programs.[5] As a matter of fact, the international philanthropic intervention during the first half of the twentieth century was so diverse that it not only promoted American and Western capitalist expansionism, it also expanded the commitment of political authorities and ideas of welfare and progress.[6]

However, the framing of several forms of technical expertise – in this case associated to state and international organizations – became not only a reference to legitimate international intervention and state policies, experts also became some sort of independent authority.[7] Humanitarian intervention and medical activism, based on ethics and action, became a wide movement in Western countries at a time of crisis and conflict.[8] As well as this, it was a matter of controversy in the US during the first decades of the twentieth century.[9] Some organizations such as the Red Cross associated the fundamental *spirit* of mercy as an essential background of the medical practice, above and beyond assessments of *moral* and political character. On the contrary, several other humanitarian associations emerged during the Interwar period not only as matter of mercy, but as a sort of activism in a time of extremes, participating in the struggle between democracy, fascism and social revolutions.[10] In that case, humanitarianism required a political involvement beyond neutrality and, to some extent, activists applied the moral imperative of humanitarian relief to go beyond the limitations of states' foreign policy and, above all, their lack of commitment to uphold democratic values, as in the case of the defence of the Spanish republic against fascism.

Recent historiography shows a wide debate about the aims and impact of the American philanthropic movement, both in the domestic domain and in the global dimension. Considered in the context of those debates, in my opinion, public health campaigns and public health experts of the RF cannot be reduced to the role of simply hidden agents of American imperialist foreign policy at a time of conflict and debate between *isolationism* and *internationalism* in American politics.[11] In addition, health politics, in the way it was promoted by the International Health Board of the RF and the Health Committee of the LNHO, contributed to improving health and living conditions in many areas and also to an increased engagement of the state administrations in the safeguard of public health. During the interwar years, international agents, or agents who had been educated at internationally leading institutions, exerted technical and ideological influence which increased the State's involvement in *health* policies, something that can be considered as a point of departure of the Welfare State policies during the Cold War era.

1 INTERNATIONAL DIPLOMACY MEETS PUBLIC HEALTH

Scientific knowledge on health is spatially situated and not something disembodied and universal. Therefore, in its production and orientation it is closely linked to the economic system and political interest.[1] It is essential to conceive science and medicine as it is made, negotiated, received and reshaped in a range of sites.[2] In the first half of the twentieth century geopolitical reasons led to a cultural and scientific hegemony, whereby social elites shaped a system of values justifying the colonial domination of the Western powers.[3] The history of international health cooperation started with the joining of forces to control communicable diseases.[4] The first initiatives and agreements on health matters among national authorities were prompted by the need of measures to protect trade to prevent the spread of pestilence – particularly cholera, plague and yellow fever.[5] Therefore, since the central decades of the nineteenth century, health occupied a relevant place in the international agenda.[6] The birth of an international sanitary movement became a reference to local policies facing the scientific and social dimensions of health and disease. It influenced the production of medical knowledge, a series of aspects of clinical practice, public health policies and campaigns, prevention and national initiatives for the health care organization in urban and rural districts.[7]

International diplomacy was the clue agent which played a prominent role in this process of international negotiation. The increasingly widespread political concern about the negative effects of health impairment over social stability also influenced the birth of an *international scientific community* around hygiene, endowed with a growing importance in the different domains, based on new forms of political and scientific legitimacy: negotiations of medical standards, the creation of national laboratories, institutes and schools of public health, sanitary campaigns, expert committees and international conferences, technical reports and sanitary interventions. The most practical uses of science and public policies were linked to the growing prestige of the expert qualification as a fundamental tool for political authorities and practical intervention.[8]

During the second half of the nineteenth century, the main sites of experimental medicine and laboratory research were research institutes, usually attached to universities, as well as national agencies that were founded in most European countries, among others, the Pasteur Institute in Paris, the Institute of Hygiene and Tropical Medicine in London, the Robert Koch Institute in Berlin, the State Institute of Health in Copenhagen and other similar ones in Madrid, Zagreb, Warsaw and Prague. These research centres were the venue of scientists around the world, particularly in the European context. Young scientists began their experimental research in fields such as physiology, serology, bacteriology or pharmacology following research programs in a widespread network.[9]

Although the scientific importance of these research institutes did not decrease during the first decades of the twentieth century, after the end of the First World War the internationalization of medical science and the increasing political and commercial importance of agreements on public health were influenced by two international organizations whose power and influence were unprecedented. The first was the Rockefeller Foundation and more particularly its International Health Board, which signed agreements with many national authorities regarding public health campaigns and designed an efficient grantees policy aiming at creating an extensive network of well-connected public health professionals.[10] The other key actor was the Health Organization of the League of Nations, which prompted an ambitious international health program by creating expert commissions, promoting international conferences, exchanging programs and experiences, promoting research in certain fields and funding health campaigns. They gave a strong impulse to vital statistics and a series of public domains such as nutrition, drug consumption, rural hygiene, standardization of diets, biological products and pharmaceuticals, maternal and child health, among others. The strategy of improving the health standards of the European population was an essential part of the international stabilization policies in a time of huge social tensions and deep conflicts.

Epidemics and Trade

Surveillance and control of epidemics were historical precedents of international intervention on health matters during the first half of the nineteenth century.[11] Maritime transport was the principal factor of plague transmission and local health committees used to apply isolation measures, quarantines and sanitary cordons. A system of clean and dirty patents had been introduced among national authorities to allow or restrict navigation depending on political interests and on the epidemic situation of the city of origin.[12] After the terrible plague that affected Marseille, in 1720, quarantine measures got more rigid in maritime stations, involving retention of the ship during a quarantine period, disinfection of goods and the medical inspection of passengers.[13] This international system of patents and the quarantine stations represent the oldest trace of international health based on a model whose main goal was preserving cities and borders from plague contagion.[14] The traditional quarantine system was closely linked to the colonial hegemony of Western powers, as a means to maintain their privileged position. A wide historiography has analyzed the role of hygiene and public health politics in the dynamics of colonialism.[15]

Feeling threatened by those national discretionary measures, several European states raised the need for international health regulations to address the spread of pandemics, with minimum damage of trade. Diplomatic contacts between governments culminated with the celebration of a dozen *International Sanitary Conferences*, whose main result was the cooperation for the establishment and implementation of rules aimed at controlling infectious diseases.[16] The Paris Conference (1851) was not the first attempt to convene international agreements on public health measures, since a long process of diplomatic action had been doing so since the early nineteenth century.[17]

To promote international agreements on quarantine regulation, the pressure of the foreign policy of the colonial powers has traditionally been considered as a key factor, mainly France and Britain, to avoid dangerous protectionist policies that could harm their commercial interests. The rise of international trade during the first decades of the nineteenth century and the commercial interests of the colonial powers were the main support to the birth of an international diplomacy for public health policies. As a matter of fact, the Sanitary Conferences were openly conceived as a political and commercial tool.

The emergence of Asian cholera, a disease seldom affecting the European societies before the beginning of the nineteenth century, appeared as a fearsome pandemic, added to the traditional epidemics, generating confusion at a crucial stage for colonial interests and the expansion of a world trade market. By the mid-nineteenth century maritime trade had increased fivefold compared to the beginning of the century. The quarantine system and other restrictive measures, implemented by the states around public health, had become a political and diplomatic tool for the fight between rival powers. In addition, epidemics were a risk for the health of the population, for social stability and for the sanitary control of ports and borders. Indeed, the Vienna Conference (1815) opened a new stage of negotiation between representatives of countries, in which international conflicts became a matter of diplomacy and negotiation rather than of war and weapons.[18]

A series of international conferences on health and demography, children's protection, tuberculosis, milk depots and venereal diseases, among others, gave way to discussions involving experts and national authorities, and international agreements on specific issues, which were apparently much more effective to fight the spread of diseases and to settle national and international policies to cope with them. In this context the international sanitary conferences were agreed as a locus of an intense diplomacy, whose interest extended beyond strictly health matters.[19]

The establishment of quarantine to prevent the spread of epidemics and regulate trade from contaminated sites was an ancient practice that had been established in many Mediterranean countries since the mid-fifteenth century. Cities traditionally had local government bodies to prevent the spread of epidemics using quarantines and sanitary cordons. After the early 1830s the preventive measures against cholera usually applied to goods and passengers coming from the Eastern countries as this was the origin attributed to the cholera plague, but they were also implemented to ships from the West Indies to prevent the spread of yellow fever. The traditional policy of quarantines and sanitary cordons was still in force at the start of the nineteenth century. Nevertheless the quarantine stations went through critical moments not only for political and commercial grounds, but also for public health arguments. Although political measures should be taken to prevent epidemics, health officers and health authorities started to discuss its usefulness. Companies associated with the import and export of products put pressure to avoid obstacles to normal trade. Sanitary cordons along land borders were even more ineffective due to fraudulent schemes of traders trying to circumvent the law to not harm their business. This controversial situation encouraged conflicts and debates, and reinforced the idea that the key issue was to establish an effective system of reporting epidemic outbreaks rather than implementing isolation and quarantine schemes. But the establishment of an effective system of recording and reporting epidemiological records required methodological agreements and a hard international coordination to ensure that the reports issued by the ports of origin were trustful and homologable, and were not handled according to pure political, military or commercial interests.

This plurality of factors made the problem of epidemics enter into the agenda of international diplomacy since the end of the eighteenth century, at a time when the pressure from big trade companies against quarantines and sanitary cordons was increasing. Moreover, economic liberalism boosted international sanitary conferences to alleviate the tendency to state protectionism.[20]

The criticism against quarantines also incorporated scientific arguments against the new doctrine of microbe contagion that justified its application, associating the origin of the disease to the environmental conditions of the endemic place where the epidemics originated. The opinion of many doctors was critical to the effectiveness of quarantine and to some arguments of the colonial medicine. As a consequence, a series of studies on the conditions of occurrence of communicable diseases was carried out to highlight the importance of sanitary and environmental local conditions apparently contributing to transform endemic into epidemic diseases, in certain regions.[21]

Under those controversial circumstances, the explosive emergence of cholera in Europe during the 1830s highly impaired the international sense of risk and impotence against new hazards. Since the sense of vulnerability increased among the Europeans, quarantine emerged as a means of trying to isolate the infectious focus, and hence to spoil the only possible mechanism of prevention.

However, the lack of certainty about the causes and mechanisms of disease transmission and the controversial diversity of opinions about routes of infection left no room for further medical and political action.

The first initiatives aiming to propose an international regulation of quarantine occurred in Louis Philippe's liberal France as an attempt to modify the previous Bourbon protectionism. As early as 1817, F. E. Fodéré advocated convening an international conference to promote agreements and regulations to end the chaos represented by the plurality of national quarantine legislations, their lack of effectiveness and the interfering commercial relations.[22] Some years later, Nicolas Chervin (1833) raised the issue again in similar terms.[23]

The growing international concern about epidemics and the controversy on quarantines opened the doors to international diplomacy. In 1834, the physician M. De Ségur-Dupeyron was commissioned by the French Ministry of Commerce to prepare a report on the various ways of implementing the quarantine system in Mediterranean ports. He made personal visits to main harbours, studied their way of implementing quarantines and reported his conclusions to the French minister.[24] De Ségur-Dupeyron established a link between trade and epidemics observing that there were no cases of epidemics in war areas where trade had been disrupted. He believed that preventive measures were necessary, but were ineffective as applied and therefore recommended the establishment of a uniform system of preventive measures, ranging from short-term quarantine until its abolition in the case of ships sailing from the Western Indies. That strategy obviously required international agreements and, despite the existence of an adverse climate for cooperation, in 1838 the French government assumed the hosting of an international conference gathering together representatives of European countries with ports in the Mediterranean Sea to negotiate a common system of quarantine and public health control of maritime routes and borders. The proposal received support from two of the largest northern European powers: Great Britain, involved in large commercial interests in the Mediterranean in transit to the Middle East and India, and Austria, affected by numerous quarantine stations on both riverbanks of the Danube and its borders with the Ottoman Empire. Participant powers aimed to generate international regulations, whereas international conferences could alleviate the difficulties of international diplomacy and move towards a peaceful resolution of political and commercial problems with a hygienic background.

De Ségur-Dupeyron's report also influenced decisions affecting other Mediterranean areas of French colonies. In 1836 a meeting was held in Tangier, attended by Dupeyron himself, which served to convene in April 1840 to all consuls of foreign states in Tangier at a meeting that was the starting point of the creation of a *Conseil Sanitaire Maritime International* in the city. The strategy of surveillance and regulation led by France, Britain and Austria was spread to other southern Mediterranean areas such as Libya, Egypt, the Ottoman Empire and, therefore, similar international health councils were created in Tunisia (1835), Constantinople (1839), Alexandria (1843) and Tripoli, which claimed some coordination and control over these strategic areas.

Although the 1848 revolution disrupted the work done in favour of international agreements around quarantine, France returned to the idea of holding an International Sanitary Conference, which finally took place in Paris (1851–2). Until the creation of the *Office Internationale d'Hygiène Publique* (1907) and the League of Nations Health Organization, a long series of international conferences on sanitary matters took place in Europe; those events becoming the most relevant open forum to discuss and negotiate international health regulations. Negotiations and agreements implied not only foreign policy, but also certain scientific concepts under debate.[25]

The first international sanitary conference took place in Paris (1851) relying on two delegates from each country, a diplomat or health authority and a medical expert. In his opening remarks, the Minister of Foreign Affairs of France noted the need to find a way of acting in accordance with the technical and industrial progress, and claimed for international harmony achieved through conferences that aimed to abolish traditional political obstacles put by local authorities to impose free trade ports and borders. Participant countries were Austria, Sardinia, Sicily, Spain, Papal States, France, United Kingdom, Greece, Portugal, Russia, Tuscany and Turkey. But the conference was definitely a failure. Only a short international agreement was signed by the representatives of a few countries such as France, Sardinia and Portugal. The Mediterranean countries were reluctant to a drastic reduction or to an abandonment of the quarantine system while France and Britain put pressure to minimize quarantines. The failure to establish a more ambitious international agreement was due to a conflict of interest between the strategy of colonial powers to facilitate maritime trade and the still prevalent public health ancestral mentality, which based prevention and control of epidemics in quarantine measures and isolation.

A second Sanitary Conference was held in Constantinople (September 1866), this time attended by thirty-one countries. France was again the main promoter proclaiming as a principal objective to take steps 'to attack vigorously the Asian cholera in its original places', rather than preventing its spread.[26] Scientific evidence based on microbiological analysis was still scarce and there was not a scientific agreement about the waterway or air transmission. The measures taken on trade surveillance and international health regulations based on quarantine were justified by public health experts to preserve Europe from epidemics, even if they negatively affected maritime traffic. A general feeling of alarm existed regarding massive pilgrimages to Mecca as well as in high-density areas like the Red Sea trade. The evident ineffectiveness of quarantine was the main point of discussion, but no alternative methods were recognized. Just a few resolutions on the expenditure of health patents by port authorities and health care control in the harbours saved the results of the Conference. As distrust predominated on the efficient management of the quarantine stations, the possibility of settling stations administered by international joint councils was an alternative. This option reinforced the geography and persistence of colonial powers generating controversy. On the other hand, debates dealt with the duration of the quarantine. Great commercial and colonial powers tried to put limits to the autonomous capacity of decision-making by the countries.

A third Sanitary Conference took place in Vienna (1874) attended by forty-four representatives from twenty countries. Given the limitations and disappointment which emerged from the Paris (1851 and 1859) and Constantinople (1865) agreements, the Vienna Conference proposed a more drastic reduction of quarantine in benefit of trade, with the opposition of health authorities responsible for maritime health and border control of some Mediterranean countries. The Vienna Conference established a distinction between land quarantine and maritime quarantine. In the first case only sanitary cordons were considered at land borders leaving each country free to adopt the most appropriate isolation measures. However, maritime quarantines were a source of great controversy when regarding the Caspian Sea and the Red Sea regions; in several ports of Europe a permanent medical inspection service was established. Disinfection and quarantine measures were implemented for just seven days in infested ports and three to seven in those under suspect.

Sometime later, the Dresden Sanitary Conference took place in 1893 convening diplomatic representation and public health delegates from Germany, Austria-Hungary, Belgium, Spain, Great Britain, Greece, Italy, Netherlands, Romania, Switzerland and Denmark. Only diplomatic delegates from Montenegro, Portugal, Russia, Serbia and Sweden-Norway attended the meeting. The predominance of diplomatic representation over public health authorities and medical experts was evident, something that also happened in previous conferences. The Conference convened by the Austro-Hungarian government established as main targets the signature of agreements to prevent obstacles to the traffic of passengers and merchandises, providing uniformity to international measures. A reform of the Health Council of Constantinople was approved, as well as an International Sanitary Board in Tehran, in accordance with the reformed model of the International Sanitary Council in Egypt. Moreover international health surveillance stations were established in the Persian frontier.

To prepare for the Conference a questionnaire for participating countries was previously distributed containing twenty-eight questions about government preventive measures, criteria for declaring suspicious a location, means of prevention, exclusion criteria and admission of goods, restrictions on certain objects, conditions and rules for disinfection, travellers retention, employee review, quarantine regime and medical checking procedures, among others. From Dresden (1893), medical inspection at ports and borders, and disinfection systems, became fundamental to go forward in the international homologation and progressive control of quarantine isolation. Indeed, quarantine stations paid more attention to medical checking as a means to control borders for the prevention of epidemics, but the new strategy involved strong investment in facilities and sanitary staff.

The International Sanitary Conference in Paris (1911) was the last milestone before the creation of the League of Nations. Germany, USA, Argentina, Austria-Hungary, Belgium, Bolivia, Brazil, Bulgaria, Chile, Colombia, Costa Rica, Cuba, Denmark, Ecuador, Spain, France, UK, Greece, Guatemala, Haiti, Honduras, Italy, Luxembourg, Mexico, Montenegro, Norway, Panama, the Netherlands, Persia, Portugal, Romania, Russia, El Salvador, Serbia, Siam, Sweden, Switzerland, Turkey, Egypt and Uruguay were the participant nations. An *International Sanitary Convention* that had been developing since 1903 was passed. Three technical commissions were established on yellow fever, pest and cholera, each commission developing an agenda to discuss scientific aspects related to causes, transmission, incubation period, symptoms, transport conditions for the contagion in maritime and land transports as a background and point of departure for prevention and disinfection. Cholera was still the main threat and source of concern.

The international sanitary movement was not an isolated initiative. It developed itself closely to national social policies along the second half of the nineteenth century. The development of liberal reformism involved a series of social changes. A particularly impotant milestone was an international meeting held in Brussels in 1853 where it was proposed to hold regular meetings with the participation of social policy makers in various countries. A couple of years later, in 1855, when the Universal Exhibition of Industry, Economy and Charitable Societies occurred in Paris, the first *International Conference on Charity* took place, insisting on the opportunity to hold regular meetings to exchange experiences and initiatives aiming to coordinate social policies. Topics such as nurseries, asylums, host institutions for abandoned children, school inspection, child labour regulations, charity kitchens, allowances for the elder, attention to the sensory deprived children, summer colonies, begging and child abandonment, charitable hospitals and home social care were some of the most important topics discussed. Those meetings represent some sort of international liberal movement trying to face poverty and marginality at a time when workers union claims and international socialism became increasingly influential and better organized.

This is the context of the first initiatives to hold international meetings on *bienfaissance,* the French version of charities. Therefore information about programs and institutions existing in various countries circulated, including their management circumstances and financial support. The first *Congrès International de Bienfaissance* was held in Brussels in 1856, thanks to the initiative of M. Ducpétiaux, Inspector General of Prisons and Charitable Institutions in Belgium, under the auspices of the King of the Belgians and the presidency of M. Charles Rogier. A comprehensive exhibition on domestic economy trying to improve housing dress of workers complemented the Conference. The minutes of the sessions and the information about different countries were gathered in a final publication.[27] A second Conference was held just a few months later in Frankfurt am Main. It received the support of political institutions such as the Chamber of Deputies in Berlin. The organizing committee of the Conference was composed by the leading groups of the liberal society: politicians, lawyers, doctors and priests from different confessions, the official languages being English, French and German. The *Congrès International de Bienfaissance* celebrated in Frankfurt was organized around three main areas: welfare, education and prison reform.[28]

The international network established during the second half of the nineteenth century by liberals and reformists seems to me an important event that has not been sufficiently taken into account by the historiography when discussing national reforms and the interaction between hegemonic and subaltern cultures.

The issues subject to consultation and the working program was extensive and covered general aspects such as welfare programs, strategies to improve the working conditions of industrial workers, charitable institutions, public schools, domestic service, protection of poor children, children's delinquency, alcoholism, compulsory education at schools, childcare institutions and also the prison system. Independently of any critical consideration, as a matter of fact these international conferences contributed an immense amount of information, which circulated between countries and created common perspectives, which then influenced the particular programs developed in different nations.

The third International Conference of Charities was held in London in 1862, on the occasion of the Universal Exhibition and the sixth meeting of the *National Association for the Promotion of Social Science*. The London Conference was organized around two major topics: the role of the State to fight children's abandonment and the universality of education and compulsory school attendance. The following conference was held in Milan in 1880, and the program covered four areas: charitable organizations, charity by almsgiving, charity hospital and healthcare and charities also lining some matter of public policy. This last section intended to discuss the model of prisons and the rehabilitation of prisoners, as well as care initiatives for abandoned children, foundling organizations and national legislative frameworks that referred to these issues. A novel aspect of the International Conference of Charities in Milan was the effort paid to encourage participating countries to report their national charitable model, the organization of health care institutions, their operations and the legislative framework.

The *Congrès International de Bienfaissance* along with the International Conferences of Hygiene and Demography (1852–1912) and the International Sanitary Conferences were the driving forces behind the international health movement during the second half of the nineteenth century. They represent an important motor driving medical and social policies in the context of liberal reformism. This movement was essential to understand the development of social statistics, public hygiene and the birth of demography. At the same time, the First International Conference on Statistics (Brussels, 1853) sought to find out the usefulness and application of statistics to the public administration, looking for the foundation for a general international service. The initiative was raised at the *Universal Exhibition on Industry* held in London in 1852. Immediately afterwards a Conference took place in Brussels (1853), followed by others held in major European cities: Paris (1855), Vienna (1857), London (1860), Berlin (1863), Florence (1867), The Hague (1869), San Petersburg (1872) and Budapest (1876). The Budapest Conference focused on issues related to demographic and health statistics. Mortality records were an important issue of discussion and the acceptance of international statistical methods to measure epidemics and to assess public health statistics was the main challenge.[29]

Parallel to the celebration of the International Conferences of Statistics, as of 1876, successive International Conferences of Hygiene and Demography took place. Several meetings took place in Brussels (1878 and 1900), Paris (1880), Turin (1882), Geneva (1884), The Hague (1887), Vienna (1891), London (1894), Budapest (1898), Madrid (1907), Berlin (1907) and Washington (1912), with an active participation of representatives from most European countries.

At the International Conference of Hygiene and Demography held in Vienna (1891), the prominent hygienist Max von Pettenkofer, one of the participants and promoter of the International Sanitary Conferences, spoke about the state of the instruction in public health in universities and medical schools. Pettenkofer was a convinced defender of the work done by the National Institutes of Hygiene in the implementation of experimental research and field campaigns to develop testing and evaluation of sanitary interventions. While acknowledging the important role of bacteriology, he highlighted that fighting infectious diseases depended more on government actions than on therapeutic technologies. He thought that hygiene and public health were to be taught at technical schools since there was a need to promote sanitary engineering, a key element for health policies in the prevention and resolution of many health problems.

The eighth International Conference of Hygiene and Demography was held in Budapest in 1894, with a wide range of topics in the agenda: etiology of infectious diseases, prophylaxis of epidemics, hygiene in tropical countries, professional and workers' hygiene, children's healthy development at school, food hygiene, urban and rural health, housing and transports. Specific sections were devoted to the Red Cross, hygiene in the army, risks and hazards, sanitary policy, gymnastics, spa establishments, veterinary medicine and pharmacy.

The ninth International Conference of Hygiene and Demography held in 1898 in Madrid and the tenth held in Paris in 1900 included similar topics in the agenda. Particular interest aroused on the children's problem related to hygiene, nutrition, schools, hospitals and prisons, unhealthy housing and disease prophylaxis, while the part devoted to demography paid attention to migrations, alcoholism and human height in relation to profession and social status.

The eleventh International Conference on Hygiene and Demography held in Brussels in 1903 summarized a series of issues that expressed most interest of public health experts and concern of authorities in the early years of the twentieth century: health of the workers, spread of infectious diseases, food hygiene, industrial hygiene, transport, colonial medicine, health statistics and alcoholism. Modernization of health facilities such as the construction of sewage systems, technologies for drinking water purification and control, urban hygiene and disinfection campaigns were also discussed. Other issues regarded occupational health like lead poisoning, fatigue and the need of rest, hygiene problems associated with textile industry, animal hair work, home-work and small industries and hygiene education in mining schools. Finally, the need of a professionalized school medical inspection as an expert body and the international coordination for comparable results of statistics on causes of death and causes of disease were the main issues. At the turn of the century the availability of updated records on health and demography was perceived as a need for medical policy and an expression of modernity and progress.

Many of the issues addressed in the International Conferences of Hygiene and Demography ended up getting attention to more specific issues, as happened with the International Conferences on Occupational Diseases, International Medical Conferences of Work Accidents and the International Conferences for the Protection of Children.

Throughout the preceding pages I have tried to discuss the multiple dimensions and strength of what could be considered an international movement on health and social interventions during the second half of the nineteenth century. It was an important part of the liberal reforms consequence of international networks. Globally considered, all these initiatives offer a general overview of the huge amount of work done during the nineteenth century in the field of public and international health, something not always recognized by current historiography. All the international events previously mentioned undoubtly created widespread networks and made a strong impulse to the creation and circulation of hegemonic forms of knowledge, which contributed to the implementation of new methods for social and medical research, putting pressure on the authorities and governments to cope with the consequences of social dominant diseases. The predominance of a preventives approach contributed to the development of social medicine and social hygiene.

Nevertheless, the first institution explicitly devoted to international health was the *Office Internationale d'Hygiène Publique* (Paris, 1907). The governments of Belgium, Brazil, Egypt, Spain, United States, France, Britain, British India, Italy, Russia, Serbia, Switzerland and Tunisia signed on 9 December 1907 in Rome an international agreement for the creation of an International Office of Public Health, whose headquarters were established in Paris.[30] The governments of the Netherlands and Portugal ratified the agreement as well and a few months later Mexico joined to the new international agency. The operating model consisted of a committee of delegates from the participant governments, whose powers were specified in an annex that included organic statute of the Office.[31]

Signatory countries were committed to participate in the operation of the Office, which declared as a fundamental principle its independence from France, despite being located in Paris. In addition, it did not have to intervene in the management of health policies by the member states. In the fourth article, the statutes declared: 'The Home Office aims to collect and disseminate among the participant states facts and documents of general interest to the public health, especially in regard to infectious diseases, especially cholera, plagues and yellow fever, proposing measures to be taken to combat diseases'.[32]

Article 6 of the agreement attached to the organic statute that created the office provided for the establishment of a Permanent International Board composed by a representative of each of the member countries. According to its statutes, the *Office International d'Hygiène* inherited the interest and concern for international coordination in border health issues that had characterized international health conferences. It exerted a permanent pressure on states to accomplish international agreements. Another main objective was the exchange of crucial information on important topics such as:

1. The general laws and local regulations in different countries in relation to communicable diseases;
2. Information on the impact of infectious diseases over the population;
3. Statistics on public health issues;
4. Information concerning sanitation projects and other public health measures taken by national sanitary administrations.

The Office began its mission with intensity, asking governments to send reports on the epidemiological situation of exotic infectious diseases, with particular reference to pest, cholera and yellow fever, as well as its presence or breakdown in colonial territories, seeking information about measures taken by national administrations to prevent their spread. Moreover, the Standing Committee of the Office requested government information about health legislation (laws, regulations, ordinances, decrees, acts, etc.) in order to publish and spread all this information, as well as reports on the general health organization and public health campaigns among the countries members of the Office, measures taken to fight communicable diseases, the organization and operation of maritime health stations and medical care organization in rural and urban areas.

The Standing Committee established, thus, a clear line of action, which incorporated two principal dimensions: firstly, international diffusion of public health policies in different countries. The *Bulletin de l'Office International d'Hygiene Publique* was the monthly publication, which summarized this information. It was written in French and served not only to collecting information, but also to put political pressure on governments to promote public health policies. During the following years until the creation of the Health Organization by the League of Nations in 1920, the *Bulletin* became the main reflection of the laws and campaigns of the states on vital statistics and epidemiological records, reflecting public health policies implemented in the member countries regarding housing, the conditions of slaughterhouses and the hygienic control of foodstuff, sewage systems and control of the quality of drinking water to avoid the dissemination of infections. The *Bulletin* included in each issue epidemiological records on mortality caused by cholera, pest and yellow fever in the various countries of the world, creating a real observatory for the prevention and fight against pandemics.

Before being relegated to a secondary role as a consequence of the creation of the League of Nations Health Organization, the *Office International d'Hygiène Publique* held two International Sanitary Conventions in 1912 and 1926 mostly focused on international regulations regarding epidemics and infectious diseases transmitted by maritime transport, quarantines, patents, sanitary passports, migrations ... mostly plague, yellow fever, cholera, typhus and smallpox. In addition it promoted a Convention on anti-diphteric serum (1930) and convened conferences on dengue and opium (1925 and 1931). The Paris Office also contributed to the improvement of health statistics and worked out surveys on tuberculosis, venereal diseases, malaria, leprosy, cancer, typhoid fever, scarlet fever, meningitis, poliomyelitis, encephalitis, goitre, medical screening, rural and urban mortality, narcotics, drinking water and modern hospitals.

With the passing of time, the President of the Health Committee of the League of Nations and several members of his committee were accepted as members of the *Office Internationale d'Hygiène Publique*. Although it did not become a part of the League after its creation, the *Office Internationale* acted in close cooperation with the Health Organization of the League, and in practice served as the general conference of the latter, i.e. drew up draft conventions, laid down general lines of policy etc. In short, it did, in the domain of health, much what the General Assembly did for the League as a whole.

A clear testimony of the collaborative actions could be found in the archives. On 2 May 1922, the head of the Health Organization of the League of Nations, the Polish bacteriologist Ludwik Rajchman issued to W. Rose, head of the International Health Board of the Rockefeller Foundation (IHB, RF) a report on the Health Organization activities developed since its creation in September 1921. He stated:

> A working agreement was arranged with the *Office Internationale d'Hygiène Publique*. Some forty Public Health Administrations of the world are represented by governmental delegates on the *Comité permanent* of this Office ... Its effective work has consisted so far mainly in the preparation of draft international sanitary conventions ... The Office however has no executive functions ... and we are to be responsible for all executive work in the domain of international public health.[33]

The policy of the Organization was formulated by the Health Committee, appointed by the Council of the League among the members of the *Comité permanent,* the *Office Internationale* and a representative of the League of Red Cross Societies and one of the ILO. Scientific, administrative and geographical arguments were taken into account for the election. The Danish serologist Thorvald Madsen was elected president of the Health Committee, the British public health expert George Buchanan Vice-President and Velghe was a member of the Committee as chairman of the Office International. The Health Committee acted through the Medical Director and the Health Section, the executive organ.

The Rockefeller Foundation and International Health

The Rockefeller Foundation was not the only philanthropic institution involved in international health activism and policies during the first decades of the twentieth century,[34] but its programs and campaigns in the US and in many foreign countries over the world marked the birth of a global conception of health more than any other organization. It was initially created in 1905 being conceived as a philanthropic institution devoted to improve agriculture and living conditions in the less developed rural communities in the United States of America, promoting culture, art and Christian values and contributing to the expansion of citizen's rights in America.[35] The initiative appeared at a time of an active American movement of scientific philanthropy. Andrew Carnegie is a prominent case when he called for the wealthy to form a commitment with the common good 'by replacing individual charity with support for systematic social improvement, which was conducive to order, productivity, and secular advancement'.[36]

With the time passing the Rockefeller Foundation designed fundamental practices and very influential principles in international health in the shaping of a global perspective through direct programs in America, as well as other specific agreements with foreign agents, such as the League of Nations Health Organization and with lots of national administrations.

The initiative to create the Rockefeller Foundation arose from Reverend Frederick Gates, a philanthropic and business advisor of John D. Rockefeller who had focused on philanthropy since 1912.[37] He thought that infectious disease and ignorance were the most important causes of poverty and exclusion. Using his influential review, Gates convinced the Rockefellers for devoting grants to set up well-funded foundations run by experts. Acting as a true visionary, he thought that modernizing medicine could have greatest impact, particularly reforming medical education, sponsoring research and helping to implement public health policies which helped to strengthen the population, eradicating infectious and weakening diseases.[38] Therefore public health and the fight against avoidable diseases became the most suitable field through which Rockefeller philanthropy could apply scientific research and technical expertise to the public good.[39]

A decade before of the philanthropic initiative the Rockefeller Institute for Medical Research was founded in New York (1901). Two years later the General Education Board (1903) was incorporated starting with a pledge from John D. Rockefeller of $1,000,000 for a ten-year plan of education 'without distinction of sex, race or creed'.[40] F. Gates was the chairman, and another prominent Baptist, Wallace Buttrick, acted first as secretary and then as president of the new institutions. In a similar way to the missions created by the Jesuits, in the sixteenth century to spread Christianity, contemporary missionaries, like those Baptists promoting the Rockefeller philanthropy as well as other members of religious groups, promoted initiatives to improve education, living conditions, health care and economic development in many areas worldwide. In the origins of the Rockefeller Foundation a combination of scientific spirit and missionary ideology converged leading to this sort of *missionaires of science and medicine.*[41]

In 1907 John D. Rockefeller had added to the initial fund for the Foundation a sum of $20,000,000. In 1909 a Rockefeller Sanitary Commission, led by Simon Flexner, was created to prepare a global report on the extent and the possibilities of cure and prevent avoidable diseases affecting American communities. The technical commission operated from 1910 to 1914. Once the report was approved, a permanent commission on health was established chaired by F. Gates and Wickliffe Rose as administrative secretary endowed with a pledge of $1,000,000 for five years.

The Rockefeller Baptist leaders considered contagious diseases, and particularly anaemia caused by hookworm disease affecting a huge population of miners, as a key factor to explain the *backwardness* of the southern states of the Union, a weakening endemic factor and an impediment for modern industrialization of wide regions of the country. Initially the project sparked controversy and opposition in the Southern regions affected, but five years later Rose acknowledged that a general recognition had arisen on the negative prevalence and effects of hookworm disease. The campaign to prevent and cure the disease was considered to be an essential part of public health work in the affected areas.[42] This campaign clearly revealed the possibilities of public health intervention.

The campaign to eradicate hookworm disease was focused on miners. It combined medical treatment with anti-helmintic pharmaceuticals, installation of latrines, promotion of shoe wearing to avoid contagion by dirty water through foot wounds and hygiene education. Following the success, the Rockefeller Foundation created the International Health Board (IHB) – reorganized as International Health Division (IHD) in 1927. During the following years and mostly along the 1920s the International Health Board exported the same scheme of sanitary intervention to other countries.

The IHD was organized around an executive staff and an advisory board settled in New York, although following its international vocation, a European office was opened in Paris and other delegations in New Delhi, Bogotá and Mexico. The association of disease and underdevelopment was the key notion which gave impulse to this particular sort of international public health philanthropy. Therefore a wide network of delegates in close relation with the national authorities drafted and financed programs helping to build and modernize health institutions and administrations. They promoted sanitary campaigns and funding schools of public health 'in North America, Europe, Asia, and South America, including Johns Hopkins, Harvard, Toronto, and Sao Paulo universities, and the London School of Hygiene and Tropical Medicine, and sponsored 2,500 public health professionals to pursue graduate study'.[43]

In the first decade of the twentieth century, the Rockefeller Institute for Medical Research, the General Education Board and the Rockefeller Sanitary Commission had been solidly established, and F. Gates, S. Flexner, W. Buttrick and W. Rose constituted the leading nucleus of the initiative, which led, at the next step, to the creation of the Rockefeller Foundation. Flexner had studied at the Johns Hopkins Medical School and spent some time visiting prominent medical and research institutions in Europe: Strasbourg, Berlin, Prague and the Pasteur Institute, coming back to Johns Hopkins, where he then transferred to the University of Pennsylvania. Buttrick had graduated at the Rochester Theological Seminar and served for twenty years in pastorates in New Haven, St Paul and Albany. Member of the executive board of the American Baptist Home Mission Society, Gates introduced him to John D. Rockefeller and he was appointed to manage the General Education Board. Buttrick recruited Rose, a professor of philosophy at Peabody College, to assume the leadership in international public health programs. This initial Baptist lobby was the nucleus that shaped and gave impulse to the new project: the Rockefeller Foundation as a worldwide philanthropic agency for ' ... the promotion of scientific agriculture, the enrichment of rural life in the United States, the development of the fine arts and the refinement of taste, the promotion of Christian ethics and Christian civilization throughout the world, the development of intelligent citizenship and civic virtue in our own country'.[44]

On the 29 June 1909, John D. Rockefeller signed a deed of trust named *The Rockefeller Foundation*, appointing three trustees: his son John D. Rockefeller Jr, his son-in-law Harold McCormick, and his influential advisor Frederick Gates. The Standard Oil Company contributed 72,569 shares valued at $50,000,000 for the explicit purpose 'to promote the well-being and to advance the civilization of the peoples of the United States and its territories and possessions and of foreign lands in the acquisition and dissemination of knowledge, in the prevention and relief of suffering, and in the promotion of any and all the elements of human progress'.[45]

When, in 1912, John D. Rockefeller Jr took control of the philanthropic policies, Gates shaped the *China Medical Board* in 1914 as a project for the expansion of Western medicine. This was his most ambitious project representing a crossroad of philanthropy, science, medicine, religion, business and imperialist global dominion.[46]

Finally the Rockefeller Foundation was officially established in 1913, after the contribution of $1,000,000 by John D. Rockefeller. Initially it was led by nine members of a committee, but soon this board gave birth to the IHB. Its founding charter declared as main principles 'the promotion of wellbeing, advance of civilization as a tool for human progress'.[47] The promotion of experimental medicine and public health international policies were to become the Rockefeller Foundation's main fields of action. Once it was decided to go beyond the limits of the American society to participate as a proactive agent in international health, its strategy, from the very beginning, consisted on establishing collaborative policies offering technical aid to national governments and health authorities to challenge public health problems, including specific campaigns against infectious diseases, grants for the instruction of experts, implementation of primary health care centres and developing public health expertise at the service of the public administration.[48]

When dealing with international interventions, the leaders of the Rockefeller Foundation were absolutely convinced of the risk of failure if campaigns were simply sponsored by agents outside the countries without any active participation and strong involvement of national and local administrations and governments. Two organs coordinated international work: the *International Education Board* and the *International Health Board*. The former promoted education and a wide range of programs of scientific research in economy, agriculture, physics and other experimental disciplines, while the latter focused on collaborative projects with governments and national health authorities on public health campaigns, advice on health care centres and training of experts in public health. Progress in public health and the improvement of health standards were considered by the RF ideologists to be founded on the expertise of public health officers, on active policies and campaigns, and the efficient role of health administrations.

In addition to campaigns against infectious diseases, such as malaria, hookworm disease and trachoma, among others requiring expertise and technical facilities, the main lines of action were directed at popularizing the principles of hygiene, instructing experts by means of national schools of public health in the frame of an international network, implementing interchange programs and grants in prominent institutions, promoting experimental research on bacteriology, preparation of sera and vaccines and the coordination of international campaigns.

In March 1910 the Senate of the USA received a bill to incorporate the Rockefeller Foundation, providing that the corporation should report annually to the Secretary of Inner Affairs on the details of its activities with a clause saying that the charter could be supervised and changed by the Congress of the USA, which, in practical terms, implied a sort of public and political control. But the bill was withdrawn by the Senate and only after a series of amendments and delays was the bill was finally passed in 1913 with a series of modifications to the original text. The total property of the corporation should be limited to an amount of $10,000,000; the income was not to be accumulated but currently applied to the purposes for which the corporation was created; after fifty years the corporation might distribute the capital and income, and after a hundred years such distribution was mandatory if decided by the Congress. The election of new trustees should be subject to disapproval within sixty days by a majority of the following persons: the President of the USA, the Chief of the Supreme Court of Justice, the President of the Senate, the spokesman of the House of Representatives and the presidents of the Universities of Harvard, Yale, Columbia, Johns Hopkins and Chicago. Finally, no more than one tenth of the maximum value of the property, held under the terms of the charter, could be invested in the securities of any one corporation. The chart was finally passed, but a huge public debate took place among the political elites along the three years of discussions in the Congress and, therefore, the figure of John D. Rockefeller became controversial and in some sense suspicious.[49]

The IHB (after 1927: IHD) was one of the first and more active organs of the Rockefeller Foundation created in 1913. Along its almost four decades of operation, the IHD was involved in activities developed in eighty countries worldwide: targeting campaigns to fight specific social dominant diseases, granting the instruction of public health officers to help the shaping of an efficient health administration and helping to develop public health facilities. After the initial hookworm campaigns priorities were put on the eradication of malaria and yellow fever, focusing as well on the instruction of public health experts at the service of national administrations.

> Under the IHD's first director, Wickliffe Rose, the organization was committed to disease eradication and control, but efforts were also directed toward the ultimate goal of educating local populations and creating sustainable public health networks that could operate independently and efficiently after the RF left a region.

> Rose's successors built upon his ideas while incorporating other strategies to combat disease. Establishing and strengthening public health institutions certainly always played a role in IHD programs, but under the tenure of Frederick Russell lab research became a priority. This change was not without conflict – it created tensions between IHD scientists working in labs and the field officers who remained abroad, delivering medical care to local populations.[50]

The public health programs promoted by the RF were predicated on the creation of both international and national professional elites of health experts as an effective and well-coordinated task force at the service of national and international health. These elites would found their expertise on statistical evidence, technical and experimental knowledge and practical training in the field to serve as authoritative references for state policies and national health services. An important element in this process – the compiling and diffusion of epidemiological information – was strongly stimulated as well by the LNHO. Following previous initiatives from the *Office Internationale d'Hygiène Publique,* since its creation, the LNHO started to collect data and circulate periodic reports that included all the European countries. We shall discuss in another chapter how, in 1921, the Organization's Health Committee set up a Service of Epidemiological Intelligence and Public Health Statistics that was devoted not only to tracking plagues, but also any infectious disease subject to compulsory notification to health authorities. Standardization of international statistical epidemiological records was the background of any future public health policy. As we shall discuss in a further chapter, the cooperation between Ludwik Rajchman, head of the LNHO, and the leaders of the IHB of the RF such as Selskar Gunn and Frederik Russell facilitated the collection of these data.[51]

The Rockefeller programs in public health followed a pattern of business efficiency, according to which, after first contact with the health authorities, a definition of the health problems to cope with and an analysis of the opportunity of a program of intervention, a specific plan was designed with measurable goals and results.[52] The plan included budgetary needs and national governments or international agencies – like in the case of the League of Nations – should assume a part of the cost, well qualified experts were appointed to run it and results should be periodically evaluated and reported to the central office through the national or regional delegates and reviewed by trustees.

After years of negotiation with a wide range of health authorities in many different countries, the IHD turned isolated international campaigns into permanent diplomatic relations with a wide range of national authorities. Its regional and national delegates cooperated with well-instructed local experts to implement their particular perspectives and approaches to eradicate health problems and to establish specific ways to institutionalize public health. The human dimension was essential in the RF pattern of work, since the main strategy consisted of the establishment of a wide network of public health experts trained as fellows, be they doctors, nurses or engineers, with the commitment of national health authorities to use them as strategic agents of medical reforms. The RF designed an elite of public health leaders perfectly connected with national and international health authorities through a perfectly drafted system of international expert networks. The already mentioned initial campaigns against hookworm disease gave fruitful experience and opened the doors to other initiatives focused on malaria and yellow fever, emphasizing an experimental and technically oriented model of public health.

Yellow fever control was one of the subsequent targets becoming one of the highest accomplishments with huge benefits for international commerce and colonial powers. In that case the virus was transmitted alongside cargo boats provoking lethal outbreaks in populations not previously exposed. The Rockefeller campaigns were implemented in endemic regions of Latin America focused on the reduction of the presence of the mosquito vector *Aedes aegypti* by means of insecticide fumigations, drainage, larvicidal fishes and preventive campaigns with a new vaccine. Max Theiler, a specialist in Tropical Medicine at the Harvard Medical School in 1930 joined the staff of the IHD of the Rockefeller Foundation, developed a vaccine against yellow fever in 1936 and became Director of Laboratories of the Rockefeller Foundation's Division of Medicine and Public Health in 1951, the same year when he was awarded with the Nobel Price for his research on yellow fever.[53]

As we shall discuss in the following pages, the scientific and social principles that guided the Rockefeller programs in international health left a huge legacy influencing the further evolution of global health and preventive medicine. They started by an identification of the problems by authorities, feasibility of the intervention according to technical and biological paradigms, budgetary support, very specific programs to guarantee efficiency and successful results, adaptation to the local conditions and the creation of international professional networks.

The Joint Program of the League of Nations Health Organization and the *Rockefeller Foundation* International Health Board/Division

The League of Nations Health Organization (LNHO) played a fundamental role in the stabilization policies during the interwar period. Public health was considered to be a main factor in this historical context due to the consequences of the war, and the postwar years, considering the negative effects of the Great Depression, huge unemployment and the subsequent deep international crisis. The LNHO was the cornerstone of international action in many fields related to health: epidemics, fight against malnutrition, campaigns against main infectious diseases – such as malaria, tuberculosis and yellow fever – and on debates and negotiations on big social problems represented by infant mortality rates and drugs consumption. In addition new targets had to be achieved, such as the definition of biological and dietary standards, the agreement on the production and compilation of epidemiological records, the international coordination of public health policies and the professionalization of expert knowledge in public health. In the process of shaping an international space in public health based on expertise as an essential reference for national and international policies, the collaboration between the LNHO and the IHB/IHD of the Rockefeller Foundation was extremely important for the analysis of situations, definition of goals and programs and the financial support to their practical implementation.

We have discussed in previous pages how international diplomacy became an essential tool not only for political stabilization, but also for negotiating solutions for most transnational health problems affecting wide regions. Commissions of experts assumed an essential role together with particular policies based on interchange programs, technical reports and international conferences of experts. All this shaped a wide network of diplomatic action around health. The expansion of systems of social and health insurance in an increasing number of States draws attention to the social and economic burden represented by avoidable diseases. The Health Organization of the League articulated an international timeline to eliminate, as far as possible, diseases considered to be avoidable or preventable.[54] The report published after one decade of activity in public health, trying to legitimate previous policies, claiming for permanence and future work, stated that: 'In all its undertakings, the Health Organization has fully observed the principle of cooperation between all nations, as laid down in the Covenant of the League. Its work responds to the universal need for the prevention of disease, which is felt more or less acutely in all countries and in all continents. It has extended its activities to all parts of the world – to the Far East and to America, to Africa and to Europe – and the results obtained during the past ten years are of good augury for the future'.[55]

The public health authorities of all countries benefited from the expertise of the International Epidemiological Service and from the expertise of the technical committees of the League. Governments could at any time request the Health Organization to place experts at their disposal to carry out specific tasks, technical reports, information or advice on specific issues. Experts' opinions were often requested to implement specific campaigns to fight against malaria, venereal diseases, dengue epidemics and many others. Sometimes policy makers requested for advice on the organization of the public health administration in certain specific fields, such as rural districts, primary health care centres or even the structure of public health administration of the whole country. Greece, Bolivia, China, Poland and Spain, among others, requested this sort of technical advice in different moments and on different issues.[56]

After the Great War many Governments had organized public health services for the implementation of active health policies, but international experts, both of the League of Nations and of the Rockefeller Foundation were convinced that much of these efforts were wrongly conceived. One of the main grounds for failure was the lack of technical expertise. They decided, therefore, to develop a diplomatic and financial strategy of cooperation with health authorities and policy makers to orient their efforts into the right direction so that preventive work and sanitary campaigns could be well planned, funded, coordinated and successfully implemented. This strategy was mainly based on the creation of an international body of expertise endowed with technical legitimacy, operating uniformly and negotiating strategies through expert commissions, technical reports and negotiating conferences, owing support of international powers and health organizations to become the essential reference of national and international health policies. In short: a global conception of public health in accordance to their own ideas. The international health diplomacy extended cooperation with other public and private international agencies, such as the International Institute of Agriculture and the International Labour Office, organizing technical expertise on nutrition, food production, occupational health and arranging interchange visits by industrial medical inspectors.[57]

The League of Nations was a complex forum of diplomatic, economic and social debates. Within the League, the Health Organization cooperated with other organs dealing with common topics of interest, such as the advisory commission for the protection and Welfare of Children and Young People, the Transit Organization and the Economic Organization and Commissions for refugees. It furnished the Opium Commission with technical advice regarding medical requirements on narcotics and reporting new drugs within the scope of the International Convention on the Traffic in Drugs.[58]

The First Assembly of the League met in November and December 1920. It decided that one session should be held every year, drafted its rules planning one yearly session, adopted rules for the administration of its budget, drew up the principles governing the relations with the Council and also decided to create the Health and Opium Committees. Initially, when the First Assembly met, the League had forty-two members. During the following decade the list of member states grew up until fifty-four including all European countries except Russia, all Latin American countries except Brazil, Costa Rica, Ecuador and Mexico; all countries of Asia except Afghanistan, Hedjaz (west of present Saudi Arabia) and Turkey and the whole Africa except for Egypt.[59] A permanent International Health Section was proposed as part of the structure of the League, to deal with serious epidemics and urgent public health problems, 'which for the sake of all countries require international consideration and standardized action'.[60] The health permanent organization would consist of an International Health General Committee, an Executive Committee and an International Health Office.

The General Committee consisted of delegates appointed by the Governments represented on the Committee of the *Office International d'Hygiène Publique*, and might include representatives of Governments not as yet signatory to the Covenant of the League of Nations, but who had signed the Convention of Rome of 1907. The Committee appointed its own President, and might at any time appoint sub-committees to consider questions of special relevance. Delegates might request the assistance of technical advisors, who could not vote and only were allowed to speak upon request by a special authorization of the President of the Committee, except if the adviser acted as deputy of a delegate who was unable to attend the meeting. Only under those circumstances they were allowed to speak and vote. As we see, very strict norms were established. In addition, the general Committee met as occasion might require, no less than once in every year, at the Headquarters of the *Office Internationale d'Hygiène Publique* in Paris. The Official languages of the International Health Section were French and English.

The Executive Committee consisted of no more than nine members of whom one acted as President of the General Committee, one a representative of the League of Red Cross Societies and one a representative chosen by the Governing body of the Labour Conference. The remaining members were elected by the General Committee among experts having technical knowledge of the Public Health Service of their own countries.

The Executive Committee elected its own Chairman and met no less than four times a year and at any time to deal with questions requiring urgent consideration. It was empowered to form sub-committees and to call in technical advisors on special points, but these advisors lacked voting power. Reports of the proceedings of the Executive Committee and of sub-committees were submitted to the General Committee. The Chairman and Members of the Executive Committee held their appointments for three years, although were eligible for re-election.

The International Health Office was settled at the Seat of the League of Nations in Geneva, appointed by the Executive Committee. The same organ appointed the *Medical Secretary,* who was responsible to this Committee for the efficient working of the International Health Office, and for any other duties assigned to him by the Executive Committee. The *Medical Secretary* had the right of direct access to the Secretary-General of the League of Nations, and was empowered to have direct communication with all Government Health Offices: what surely made him a key figure and probably the most relevant person within the scheme of the health organization of the League. He was entitled to attend all meetings of both Executive and General Committees, and was a member ex-officio of all Committees. The Staff of the International Health Office at the seat of the League of Nations was appointed by the Executive Committee on the recommendation of the Medical Secretary, consisting of persons of different nationalities as far as possible with regard to the efficiency of the work of the Office.

The Headquarters of the International Health Office was at the headquarters of the League of Nations in Geneva. As the health organization of the League acquired stability a process of negotiation for the integration of the *Office International d'Hygiène Publique* did start. Initially the new International Health Organization wanted to get integrated under the direction of the League of Nations, but retaining its existing establishment in Paris.[61] Accordingly the Bureau of the *Office International d'Hygiène Publique* would undertake new duties assigned to it by the Executive Committee, in accordance with the resolution agreed to by the Committee of the *Office International d'Hygiène Publique* at the meeting held in Paris on 30 October 1919. Nevertheless, both agencies had different financial schemes and responded to different objectives. The expenses of the new Organization and the International Health Office of the League of Nations were to be paid from the Consolidated Funds of the League and conversely the expenses of the *Office International d'Hygiène Publique* were paid as before by contribution of the member States, according to the appointment of the Rome Convention.

The International Health Office had to advise the League of Nations in matters affecting health, as its principle duty. Due to the international dimension of the League, the Office commitment was bringing into closer relationship with each other the administrative health authorities of the different countries, organizing programs to improve easy interchange of information on matters where immediate preventive measures against disease had to be taken. It also provided a ready organization for securing internal agreements and for administrative action in matters of international health. It was particularly helpful for examining those subjects proposed before the executive committee and the General Committee to make a final decision, with a view to the conclusion of International Conventions. As a sort of coordinating organ in matters of international health, the Health Office was to be advisory to the International Labour Office on questions related with health, and give advice and expertise to the League of Red Cross Societies and other voluntary organizations.[62]

The Executive Committee was empowered to draw up new Conventions that had to be submitted to the General Committee for consideration and approval.[63] Any Convention agreed to with other agencies had to be signed by the President of the General Committee and the Medical Secretary of the International Health Office. In September 1921 the Second Assembly of the League set up a Health Organization and created a Health Section of the permanent secretariat as its executive organ. This was one of the three technical organizations of the League. The President of the Committee, the Danish Thorvald Madsen, was a bacteriologist Director of the State Serum Institute in Copenhagen, and several members of the Committee belonged to the *Office International d'Hygiène Publique.* The director of the Health Section was the Polish Ludwik Rajchman, public health expert with previous experience in the Polish health administration, former director of the National School of Hygiene in Warsaw.[64] This elite constituted the leading nucleus of the public health policy and social medicine designed and promoted by the League of Nations during the interwar years.

The Health Organization of the League's Secretariat was created by the Third Assembly in 1922, substituting the Health Committee previously appointed in 1921. Previously article 23 of the covenant of the League of Nations had foreshadowed some sort of institutional health work when it stated: 'the members of the League will endeavour to take steps in matters of international concern for the prevention and control of disease'.[65] The demographic catastrophe and the impairment of the state of health of the population after the Great War claimed for political measures, overwhelming the capacity of the states. Under dramatic circumstances in the second session of the Council a decision was made to convene an International Conference of Health Experts to draw up a scheme for the Health Organization.

The League, similar to the Rockefeller Foundation in previous years, became aware of the importance of health as subject for international concern in 1920, when typhus and relapsing fever were pandemic in Eastern Europe and represented a threat for the rest of the Continent. The situation overflowed any possible control by the health administration and policy makers of the national governments involved and the League, as an emergency measure, set up an Epidemic Commission with headquarters in Warsaw. The extremely serious threat opened the first contacts between the LNHO and the RF and paved way for the consolidation of the Health Organization as a permanent body of the League. Notwithstanding, when the resolution calling for its creation was first presented to the Assembly for approval, its provisional character was emphasized. A general concern about the proliferation of inner bodies advised the League to be cautious. And a budget on a fixed basis of 1,000,000 SF yearly was adopted. The same amount yearly was approved during the following years and the HO consolidated its meaningful role in the frame of the League activities.

The conversations between the LNHO and the RF started as soon as 1920, as a consequence of the critical pandemics affecting regions in Poland and Russia, immediately after the Health Organization had been established. In February of 1920, Wickliffe Rose, head of the IHB of the RF, sent a letter to George E. Vincent, President of the RF IHB enclosing a copy of a proposed health scheme for the League of Nations.[66] Ludwik Rajchman had previous experience of collaboration with the RF and the international activities of the IHB were known and estimated by the HO leaders. In addition the financial situation of the HO was never in accordance with the demands of intervention to palliate the endless serious health problems.

In March 1922, after conversations between Rajchman and Rose, a proposal of collaboration was presented to the IHB of the RF consisting of a five year aid program mainly devoted to develop an International Epidemiological Intelligence Service on a more efficient basis, to make it so useful and indispensable to national governments that they would fund it after the five years. A second target was to develop a scheme for international exchange of public health experts engaged in health policies at national administrations. The Rockefeller IHB approved this initial project and authorized the required funds to start with. An international consensus around the political importance of health and the necessity of expertise had emerged. Therefore experts reached great political influence. The ideology under these philanthropic agreements could be summarized in these words taken from a letter from Rose to F. F. Russell:

> There are certain health functions that are essentially international in character; national governments cannot undertake them; they are important for the health of the people of all lands. The League is the first agency to be created that can undertake them. We should like therefore to see the Health Organization of the League succeed. For this reason the Board has shown disposition to aid in getting itself established. The Board stands ready to serve if and when such service may seem desirable and feasible.
>
> Quite regardless of what may have happened in the past, the officers of the International Health Board would not be disposed to commit the Board to expenditures for any program of the League until the Health Committee has endorsed it as sound and is prepared to back it wholeheartedly. The scheme is theirs, not ours. They must make up their own mind about it in their own way.
>
> Please understand that we are in full sympathy with Health Organization of the League; that we regard it as having opportunity to perform a number of public health functions which are tremendously important to the wellbeing of people of all lands and which no other agency can undertake.[67]

Rose's words express clearly the real grounds and late interests of the RF when accepting collaboration with the League on public health programs. It seems that the opportunity of an agreement was under no question and both sides were aware of the mutual benefits. On 18 November 1921 Rajchman sent a report to the RF entitled *The League of Nations Health Organisation: What it is and How it Works*.[68] He informed the RF that the Genova Conference, devoted to the economic reconstruction of Europe, had to decide whether the anti-epidemic campaign in Eastern Europe was to be conducted by the League Health Organization. This was one of the recommendations of the recently celebrated Warsaw Health Conference, which furthermore insisted on the urgent necessity for a large-scale campaign against epidemics in Eastern Europe as an indispensable preliminary to the work of economic and social reconstruction. The hazard represented by out-of-control epidemic diseases was perceived as a huge obstacle, and it overcome a *condition sine qua non*. It is worthwhile to retain that all the nations represented at the Genova Conference, including Germany and Soviet Russia, were also represented at the Warsaw Conference.

Since December 1921 the Health Committee of the League had organized an Epidemiological Intelligence Service [EIS], in order to inform all national health authorities rapidly and effectively of the incidence of epidemic diseases. The need of such a central clearing house for epidemiological information had long been felt and was particularly acute in view of the pandemics affecting Eastern Europe after the Great War. The *Monthly Epidemiological Intelligence Bulletin* contained statistics and charts on the incidence all over the world of cholera, typhus, relapsing fever, dysentery, smallpox, anthrax, scurvy and other transmissible diseases. Notwithstanding the existence of such initiative, methods of recording, systematization and coordination of statistical information required further development.

In December 1921, the Health Organization convened a Conference in London. This time epidemics and epidemiology records were not the topic of discussion. Another important issue emerged and needed negotiations and agreements: the standardization of sera and serological tests, as the starting point of a general inquiry undertaken conjointly with the *Office International d'Hygiène Publique.*

The various systems of measuring and testing the strength of anti-toxins had evolved independently of one another within different nations and even by different doctors of the same nationality, thus causing much confusion and many difficulties and conflicts. The creation of an international platform to negotiate a uniform system of units of measurement for drugs, sera, vaccines, vitamins, hormones and other biological products appeared as a necessary piece of international cooperation that only an organization such as the League Health Organization could undertake. The National Institutes of Hygiene and the Serological Institutes of Austria, Belgium, France, Germany, Great Britain, Italy, Japan, Poland, Switzerland and the United States took part in the London Conference. The Conference elaborated a program of enquiry and research, to be carried out under coordination by the different national laboratories, and centralized and coordinated by the Copenhagen State Institute, acting as a clearing house for all the standardization work. Participants agreed that the results of this first program of coordinated research had to be examined and further conclusions adopted at another conference to be held at the Pasteur Institute in Paris.

The international health program, drafted initially by the League of Nations, which was immediately presented by Ludwik Rajkmann to the RF was seen very positively by the Rockefeller authorities. Rose ended his assessing report with the following words:

> it may be said concerning the program as a whole that in performing this humanitarian service the League is bringing the nations together in a field where each has all to gain and nothing to lose; where without conflict of interest the spirit and technic of cooperative effort may be demonstrated and learned. The mutual understanding and good-will thus created will stand the League in good stead when it comes to deal with the vastly more complex and difficult problems involved in international politics and economic competition.[69]

At the beginning of September Eric Drummond informed Rose that the Council of the League of Nations, at its meeting of 2 September 1922, had passed a Resolution inviting the Health Committee to consider the administration of the funds placed by the Rockefeller Foundation for the purpose of developing the Epidemiological Intelligence Service (EIS) and instituting an Interchange of Public Health Officials between various countries.[70]

Following previous contacts, Drummond, a British diplomat and the first Secretary-General of the League of Nations, sent to Rajchman the letter received from Rose, sent the 14th June 1922, in which he stated that the Executive Committee of the IHB of the Rockefeller Foundation, at its meeting on 12 June 1922, authorized the officers of the board to enter into an arrangement with the Health Organization of the League of Nations for the maintenance of an International Interchange of Public Health Personnel on an international scale for a period of three years beginning 1 October 1922, and for this purpose to commit the Board for a sum not exceeding 60,000 dollars for any one year.[71] Rose also suggested the formulation of an agreement between the League of Nations and the Rockefeller Foundation including support to the IES.[72]

The Agreement was made between the League of Nations, acting through its Secretary-General, and the Rockefeller Foundation, acting through the Executive Committee of the IHB. Initially it dealt with the maintenance of an International Interchange of Public Health Personnel on an international scale since October 1922 and to continue for no less than three years. The program of the Interchange of Public Health Personnel was conducted along a series of general lines: to bring public health administrators in different countries into closer relationship with each other, to make comparative examination of the organization and the legislation related with public health in different countries and to obtain the cooperation of the public health administrations in different countries to agree upon a uniform standard of public health and similar regulations. Initially the program was conceived on grants towards the expenses of sending from time to time a number of public health officials from different countries to discuss and learn about a specific topic. The interchanges of experts could give opportunities of exchanging views on health problems and have options of acquainting themselves with the public health organizations of those more developed countries with the manner in which the regulations, facilities and strategies were applied, and with the duties of the health officials in different nations. Annual reports done by the administration of the Interchange of Public Health Personnel program were to be rendered to the Council and Assembly of the League of Nations, and copies of these reports were to be forwarded regularly to the International Health Board of the Rockefeller Foundation. Thus both institutions established a control mechanism for an assessment of the results obtained.

This initial proposal by the Health Organization of the League of Nations was amplified by the RF, including the study of the simplest and most reliable methods of obtaining information regarding the incidence of disease and the progress of epidemics, as well as implementing comparative studies of public health statistics in different countries and the world distribution of particularly meaningful diseases. The publication and spread of special reports and periodical bulletins, made available for any administration, were included as an essential target, a necessary point of departure for an assessment of the public health situation in the world.

The Rockefeller Foundation agreed to pay an annual subvention to meet the expenses of the interchange of public health personnel and the improvement of an international epidemiological intelligence service for three years between 1922 and 1925. The Financial Director of the Secretariat of the League of Nations was the manager of the subvention paid by the Rockefeller Foundation as a separate fund audited, as directed, by the Council of the League of Nations. The agreement included an annual statement of account rendered to the Council and Assembly of the League of Nations. Copies of these statements were to be forwarded regularly to the IHB of the RF. The Agreement was approved by the Council of the League of Nations and passed to the IHB of the RF. In accordance to it, the Budget for 1922 was:[73]

Total Appropriation			392,125
Health Committee			63,000
Special Enquiries and Investigations			63,000
Salaries:			178,500
	Medical Director	52,500	
	Assistant Medical Officer	31,500	
	Assistant Medical Officer	25,200	
	Assistant Technical Officer	25,200	
	Technical Assistants	21,000	
	Technical Clerks, Draftsmen and Secretaries	23,100	
Travelling, Removal and Vacation			
Expenses of Secretariat			31,500
Printing, Publishing, etc.			26,625
Cables, Telegrams &c. (For Epidemic Notifications)			21,000
Miscellaneous			11,500

Table 1.1: **The International Health Organization Budget for 1922 (Swiss Francs). Rockefeller Archive Centre, NY.**

Salaries	One Technical Officer	22,000
	Two Members of Section	27,400
	Two computing Clerks	18,000
	One Draughtsman	9,000
	Publications	23,600
	Cables	21,000
		121,000
Scheme for a Five Year Period:		1,426,000
Annual Appropriation:		285,200

Table 1.2: **Epidemiological Intelligence Service (Budget for 1922). Rockefeller Archive Centre, NY.**

For the operation of the scheme on *Interchange of Public Health Officials*, it was approved to hold four times a year a monthly workshop at which fifty Medical Officers of Health commissioned by ten to fifteen Governments would be addressed by six leading sanitarians. The Medical Officers would then proceed to work within the ranks of another Public Health Administration for a further period of eight weeks. This was the budget:

I. Fifty Medical Officers		
	Subsistence Allowance 25 SF/day/30 days	37,500 SF
II. Six Teachers		
	Subsistence Allowance 70 SF/day/30 days	12,600 SF
	Four Courses in Twelve Months	200,400 SF
II. Grants towards travelling expenses of Medical Officers from low exchange countries, as well as travelling expenses of teaching staff		100,000 SF
		300,000 SF

Table 1.3: **Interchange of Public Health Officials (Budget for 1922). Rockefeller Archive Centre, NY.**

Once these first steps were overcome and the first initiatives put in place – including the agreements with the Rockefeller Foundation IHB as a nuclear part – the scheme for a *Health Organisation of the League of Nations* was drawn up in May 1923 by the members of the Health Committee of the League together with the delegates of the *Comité Permanent de l'Office International d'Hygiène Publique* (OIHP). The approval was passed at the fourth Assembly in September 1923 and the structure consisted of a Health Committee, Advisory Council and a Health

Section. The Health Committee was composed by some twenty members, chosen between prominent medical specialists and officials in charge of public health services in several countries. Those experts were selected according to their technical qualification, belonging to various countries in Europe, Latin America and the Far East, out of any Governmental representation. On the principles of the new institution it was emphasized that their scientific opinions should not be conditioned by any political consideration, since both the Health Committee and the Health Organization were not political bodies. In addition, some of the members did not belong to member countries of the LN, one of them being the head of the Federal Health Service of the United States of America.

The chart stated that the members of the HC should meet twice a year, their principal duty being to lay down the program of work for the Health Section, as well as giving expert advice on technical questions regarding health and disease submitted to the Committee by the Council and the Assembly of the LN.[74] Since its creation, the HC was conceived as being assisted by technical committees and by the conclusions of conferences of experts, two main working instruments very common in the dynamics of the League of Nations.

The Advisory Council was appointed by the *Comité Permanent de l'Office International d'Hygiène Publique* (OIHP), and the Health Section was an executive organ, being an integral part of the League Secretariat composed by some fifteen public health experts, epidemiologists and statisticians of several nationalities who carried out the program drawn up by the Health Committee. It made a task of coordination among different committees, collecting and spreading information, making preparations for conferences, publications and translations, connecting research groups of experts and establishing bridges among the different agents; a networking activity which was essential for the success of the institutional pattern.

The Health Organization established a series of methods of work consisting of the establishment of committees of experts coordinating work on the field; undertaking laboratory research in the various national and international institutes and laboratories; summarizing documentary and bibliographical information; and pursuing epidemiological and medico-social enquiries by means of missions, campaigns and technical reports. There were also committees of Government representatives dealing with matters requiring the close collaboration of national administrations and health services. The Health Organization used to convene international conferences not only to face the most relevant threats for international or regional health, but also to develop technical approaches and promote agreements helping to internationalize standards of several types.[75]

One of the most common patterns employed by the Health Organization for the international coordination of scientific matters was to summon a committee of experts to discuss the issue concerned and draw up a proposal of an intervention program. The investigations were then spread among a series of prominent scientific institutions whose representatives could assess the content and propose variations into the program and plan of action. Sometimes the directors of those institutions met regularly and when they had completed their task, then a final meeting was held at which a joint report was prepared embodying their findings. This was the procedure frequently used by expert commissions such as the ones for standardization of biological products, nutrition, malaria, mother and children protection and epidemics. Sometimes expert committees carried out enquiries on the field and went to different countries to compare methods of managing specific issues, to discuss health care models, learn about the efficiency of certain sanitary campaigns etc. Exceptionally the League even established its own laboratory in Central Africa for the use of the research committee, but the norm was to appoint a single researcher or attach one of its experts to an already existent scientific mission in the concerned country.

Which were the guiding principles, which governed the Health Organization activities? Indeed the great diversity of problems it had to deal with required a plurality of methods of approach, depending on the nature of the problem to cope with. Nevertheless some general principles were implicit in its way of operating. First the Health Organization devoted its work to solve practical problems without any sort of involvement in pure scientific research. In addition, it dealt with practical health problems only if they had an international dimension. This international character could derive either from the nature and extent of the countries affected, or from the international condition of the required research or sometimes from the international coordinating measures required, as in the prevention of and fighting against famine or serious epidemics.

Only in the case that a Government requested technical advice or assistance the principle of internationality could be set aside, if the demands were in accordance with the orientation of the HO specialized work. Epidemics, famine, rural hygiene, malaria, children and mother's health, were some of the topics on which several countries demanded advice and expertise from the Health Organization.

The Health Committee was composed of high representatives of public health services and public health experts in several countries. The plurality of the issues and the technical dimension of the strategies of intervention as activities started to spread, making it convenient to distribute the work among members and to turn over some cases to specialists. The Committee, therefore, decided to establish several commissions devoted to challenge the main social diseases and health problems. Those experts' commissions were devoted during more than two decades of activity of the League to malaria, sleeping sickness, tuberculosis, cancer, smallpox and vaccination, leprosy, rabies, infant mortality and child welfare, trachoma, standardization of biological products and nutrition. Other *ad hoc* commissions dealt with cooperation between insurance organizations and public health services, working together with other organizations of the League of Nations and with Public Health Authorities of various countries.

In 1926, a long memorandum sent to the central New York office of the RF by Selskar Gunn, showed a positive assessment of the role developed by the Health

Organization during its first years of work.[76] According to Gunn's assessment, the evolution of the Health Organization program of work had followed three stages. First, when the Health Section was organized (1921–2) general doubt prevailed as to whether it would be possible to demonstrate the utility of international health work and whether it would be forthcoming from the public health services in the different countries of the world. More than financial support, moral and political support was the decisive factor at this stage. In this initial stage, the program of work, the list of activities and the several initiatives were taken, to a large extent, by the members of the Health Section. When the first results were achieved, particularly in regard to Biological Standardization, Epidemiological Intelligence Service and the Interchange of Public Health Officers, the Health Committee were encouraged to take a lead and, at the second stage, its initiative and responsibility increased. After two years of the Section work, sanitary administrations of several governments came to appreciate its usefulness and at the third stage (*c.* 1926, the date when the memorandum was written by Gunn) they began to apply to the League for advisory opinions, for the creation of special commissions or for the investigation of public health problems of particular importance.

The Assembly attitudes regarding the Health Organization corresponded basically to these three stages: first, constant references were made to overlapping work with the *Office International d'Hygiène Publique.* After two years a scheme of Organization was adopted and the usefulness of the activities were recognized although great difficulties were still found in the budget commission, which was always restrictive. But the in the following two Assemblies even this obstacle was removed. In 1925, a strong pressure in the Health Budget on the part of the British Government was finally accepted and increased to one million SF.

Both the general program of work and the budget of the LN have been placed on a stable basis, not only by the League's own budget but also by Grants of the IHB RF which amounted in 1926: $128,840 exclusive for the Singapore Bureau and a total of $154,000. Rajchman explained that the appropriations in the League's budget made it possible to maintain a nucleus of the EIS and continue, although on a reduced scale, the interchanges. Credits for the consolidation of the Singapore Bureau had been essential and publicly recognized at the January session of the Advisory Council at Singapore.

At this stage, Rajchman's strategy consisted of obtaining the collaboration of the best-qualified workers, sometimes not easy to recruit for the League. Good medical training, university distinctions, administrative experience in public health and knowledge of languages, as well as certain diplomatic skills: this was the ideal profile. Gunn was fully aware in 1926 of the technical competence of officers from various nationalities, including British, American, French and German who could get involved as members of the Health Section.

Thus the continuation of the IHB grants was considered to be not only essential, in order to allow of the stabilization of the Section activities, but also to preserve the technical team of public health workers responsible for the executive activities of international public health work. The work of the Health Section was considered by the RF leaders to be a systematic effort to use public health activities for the promotion of closer understanding between the various governments of the world; that is to say, for an international policy of stabilization. The LN was not to get engaged in laboratory research or put its main effort on stimulating scientific discoveries, but its scope as a public health international organization was to spread as much as possible the practical application of the results as it was in consonance with the program of the national health administrations.

According to the first signed agreement, grants from the Rockefeller IHB – with the exception of funds for an epidemiological bureau settled at Singapore – were to finish in 1927. The uncertain future for the years coming meant that medical officers paid out of the grants must be informed on whether or not their contracts would be renewed. In September 1927 the League's budget had to be passed, but the budget by the Financial Commission was previously approved in April–May. This crucial matter was the first topic to be discussed by Gunn with the President of the RF and the Director General of the IHB upon his arrival in New York.[77]

Just before this occurred, Selskar Gunn expressed to F. Russell his satisfaction:

> You yourself are about as familiar with the work of the Health Section of the League of Nations as I am. In general it seems to me that considering the relatively short period of time, which was elapsed since its creation, it has done remarkable work both from the point of view of quality and quantity. No doubt there are matters subject to criticism, but it seems to me that, taken all in all, the results obtained have been distinctly noteworthy. In my own travels in Europe I have heard nothing but praise of the work of the Health Section of the League of Nations.[78]

The general policy traditionally followed by the RF in its international programs of cooperation with national authorities was to limit the period of aid to five years, leaving its further development to the expenses of the targeted country involved. But, in this case, the leaders of the IHD considered a five-year period to be insufficient. With an organization of the complexity of the LN, it was hardly to be expected that in five years the difficulties could had been overcome; therefore Gunn called for an extension considering that the League representative Ludwik Rajchman was not so keen to initiate new activities, but rather to stabilize those already initiated. 'If you should be in agreement with Dr Rajchman's proposition, it would mean that in 1927 a total of $158,820 would be necessary, including the $50,000 for Interchange. In 1928 $143,820 including 25,000 for interchange and on a five-year basis, there would be needed $118,820 per year'.[79]

According to Strode's *Memorandum*[80] the one million Swiss francs which the Health Organization received annually represented approximately 4 per cent of the League's entire budget and 6.6 per cent of the budget of the Secretariat. The distribution of funds of the Health Organization for 1927 and 1928 was as follows:

Activity	*Expediture 1927 (Swiss Francs – SF)*	*Expediture 1928 (SF estimated)*
Epidemiological, Public health, Medical Intelligence, Statistics and Documentation (including Singapore Bureau)	674,200	633,900
Health Committee	55,700	66,340
Standardization serological and Biological products. Including Nomenclatures causes of death and morbidity statistics	57,200	123,300
Technical Missions, Conferences and enquiries	279,000	276,200
Interchange Public Health Staff	480,000	500,600
General and Miscellaneous	175,000	207,000
TOTAL AMOUNT:	1,721,100	1,807,340

Table 1.4: **Rockefeller Foundation Funds for the Health Organization of the League of Nations Joint Program (1927–8). Source: G. K. Strode, *Memorandum on The Health Organization of the League of Nations and the Relationship thereto of the International Health Division of the Rockefeller Foundation*, Rockefeller Archive Centre, NY.**

The combined expenditures and pledges made by the Rockefeller IHD to the Health Organization began in 1922 and were supposed to amount until 1934 a total of $1,234,487.07, according to Strode estimations.[81] The peak of IHD aid was in 1925 amounting for $165,004.90, and from 1925 to 1934 the IHD pledges decreased gradually until $22,400 in the last year.[82]

The percentage relationship of the IHD grants to the HO budgets was:

	Rockefeller percentage relationship to Health Organization estimate	Far Eastern Bureau estimate
1924	43	—
1925	31	100
1926	40	63
1927	35	55
1928	34	43

Table 1.5: **Percentage Relationship of the Rockefeller Foundation grants to the Health Organization Budgets. Source: G. K. Strode, *Memorandum on The Health Organization of the League of Nations and the Relationship thereto of the International Health Division of the Rockefeller Foundation*, Rockefeller Archive Centre, NY.**

The following table represents the summary of the first decade of collaboration:[83]

	Operative from	Duration	Type
Grant I:			
Interchange of public health officers			
	1923	3 years	Fixed
	1926	3 years	Decreasing scale
	1929	3 years	Fixed
Grant II:			
Epidemiological Intelligence & Statistics	1923	5 years	Fixed
Epidemiological Intelligence & Documentation	1928	7 years	Decreasing scale
Grant III			
Singapore Bureau	1925	5 years	Decreasing scale

Table 1.6: **Rockefeller Foundation Funds for the Health Organization of the League of Nations Joint Program (1922–30). Source: G. K. Strode, *Memorandum on The Health Organization of the League of Nations and the Relationship thereto of the International Health Division of the Rockefeller Foundation*, Rockefeller Archive Centre, NY.**

After six years of financial support, Ludwik Rajchman proposed the Rockefeller Foundation to enlarge the collaboration period.[84] The internal documentation of the RF shows how George E. Vincent wondered if Rajchman could control the Committee and prevent it from playing active politics. The Rockefeller leaders wondered about the attitude of the League as a whole and they thought about the idea of implementing small grants for brief periods; the same as what they had previously done for the instruction of public health experts of a series of countries worldwide. They feared that a long plan for seven years could be under political pressure. Russell transmitted the idea that there was an agreement on the continuity of the Singapore Bureau after the RF financial support, as well as to continue with studies in public health administration and coordinating programs for public health schools. The interchanges program received very positive comments from Russell.[85]

The IHD of the Rockefeller Foundation was concerned about national problems carrying out its cooperation work with national departments of health, bringing international experience to national problems, but not dealing precisely with health problems of an international dimension.[86] When a national problem had an international dimension, the IHD tried to establish a cooperative program with all nations involved, on a national basis, and not by international cooperation, contributing a common perspective and a common method of approach. The yellow fever and hookworm intervention campaigns were designed according with this pattern. The respective fields of the IHD and the league were defined by Russell:

> The IHD should attempt to do what the League can never be expected to do such as studies in local health organization and administration and local surveys in which the IHD may furnish personnel and a part or all of the budget. The League can, of course, give valuable advice on general principles and the organization of the central offices. We can manage surveys and experimental county health organizations.[87]

The plans of the LNHO for further extensions in international health were set in January 1928 around the following issues:

> a) New activities of the Eastern Bureau in Singapore. The Asian Bureau was expected to act as a general agency for all the activities of the Health Organization and not only as a locus for epidemiological records, working out as well special lines of research of interest for the Eastern countries.
>
> b) Studies in public health administration models, with a special attention to existing and future relations between health insurance organizations and public health services. Maternal and infant mortality, tuberculosis, venereal diseases, malaria … and other infectious diseases were also mentioned as subject of research. High mortality and high morbidity were matter of concern. Moreover, an international coordination of the instructive programs and activities developed by national schools of public health and national institutes of hygiene required specific action.
>
> c) Extension of the interchange of experts program including practical training in the field, public health activities in various fields, preventive campaigns, specialists' instruction, joint research and international surveys. All of them were the basis for an international community of public health experts under the guidelines of the RF and the League.[88]

Rajchman expected from the IHD the funds needed for the implementation of these activities, which amounted $180,000 to $280,000 to cover a seven-year period. But the answer of the IHD of the RF was cautious and prudent. The IHD leaders considered that the proportion of their contribution to the total budget should not be increased but rather diminished because '… there might be a serious reaction if the Health Section were to come to be regarded as an adjunct of the Rockefeller Foundation'.[89] Fears at the accusation of manipulation and desire for control the international health policies of the League according to the Rockefeller interests made the American foundation more cautious. Obviously the RF wanted the Singapore Bureau's activities to follow, but considered that the budget should be mostly funded by the regional governments involved. Therefore in 1928 the RF denied new grants to put pressure on national governments. On the other hand, some discussions arose within the Rockefeller IHD around the participation in a coordinated program for schools of public health, since these institutions were considered to be national affairs. As a matter of fact, the orientation and programs in the national schools were determined by national considerations and maybe national authorities were not interested on international cooperative agreements. But the IHD was highly interested in continuing support to the negotiation on biological and pharmaceutical standards, something closely related not only to the expansion of scientific research, but also to the health industry and financial profit.

The reaction of Rajchman to the initial objections raised by the RF to the continuity of the collaborative programme expressed great disappointment.[90] He claimed for a firm commitment to the IHD, considering the importance of continuity for those programs to be successful. He showed his expectancies to be able to rely on some stable financial collaboration from the RF International Health Division for the following years. However, following previous patterns of collaboration, the IHD preferred to consider new projects and to negotiate new subventions, instead of extending old programs. On the contrary, Rajchman sustained that if new grants to the previous programs were not contemplated, any activities would have to be reduced drastically. In the case of the interchange of public health experts – a project that will be discussed in a further chapter – since the program had been extended to extra-European countries, the appropriation of the whole program by the League was not sufficient to cover it.[91] As a consequence of this process of negotiation finally the grant attributed by the RF to the League – previously 150,000 SF per year – was increased in 1928 from other items in the League's health budget to meet a program of two European and one Indian collective interchanges, although other programs for individual scholarships were severely reduced. Notwithstanding it was previewed that in three years' time even this limited program would have to come to an end if financial conditions would not improve.

Similarly, the periodical publications of the International Epidemiological Intelligence Service – Weekly and Monthly Epidemiological Reports, an Annual Epidemiological Review and the International Health Yearbook – had considerably increased the amount of information made available. Moreover the statistical surveys and field studies directed to new fields of research and morbidity statistics, all were widely extended. The continuity of epidemiological information as well as the need for arranging conferences, technical meetings etc. would have suffered considerably in the case funds were not sustained.

Something similar happened to the Singapore Bureau, which was indeed acting as a sort of general agency of the Health Organization in the Far East region, but the local government's contributions and the League of Nations funds could not afford the continuity of all functions previewed. Japan, India and Australia made meaningful contributions, but governmental funds were subject to parliamentary vote and this created uncertainty and lack of stability about future plans and stable budget. Due to this unsteady situation, a reserve fund had been created by the League for the Singapore Bureau, but the threat of withdrawal of the RF grants raised serious problems to the continuity and legitimacy of the international public health programs implemented by the Health Organization of the League. The long and reflexive memorandum prepared by G. Strode emphasized the importance of the work done, its consequences and the opportunity of supporting a further agreement:

> The Health Organisation has now reached a stage of its development when the sanitary administrations of practically all the countries of the world are looking to it for collaboration and advice. For example studies in leprosy have been seriously taken up at the insistent request of Latin-American and Far-Eastern administrations. Programs for anti-tuberculous measures are being worked out for certain new countries at their request. Certain Latin-American republics are sending their principal health officers to Geneva for long periods; in one instance for the purpose of elaborating the reform of the entire sanitary and medical organisation of the country. The most promising field of coordinating effort between the public health services and the health insurance organisations has only just begun. The possibility of coordinated studies being undertaken on our initiative by the new schools of public health and the leading Institutes of Hygiene and Medical Research is being opened up. The very important problem of nutrition is ripe for international study and the active participation of the Medical Research Council of Great Britain and the leading biochemists of Germany, Switzerland and the Scandinavian countries is already assured, but cannot possibly be undertaken within the limits of the present budget, even if the Foundation's share is also stabilised at the present figure.
>
> Indeed, the Section's work has reached a stage when a definite program of activity must be elaborated for a considerable number of years and systematically prepared. This involves not only preliminary surveys, and studies, but also the preparation of the necessary competent personnel. In addition, it will be realised that an official international health organisation must have a considerable margin for unforeseen developments arising out of the ever increasing suggestions emanating from the public health services and from the Government, as well as such emergencies as the recent earthquake in Bulgaria.
>
> In this connection, the very obvious need for a close understanding with the IHD must again be emphasised, namely as to its future programme of work, and its policy for a number of years to come. Both organisations are operating in the same field and as often as not in the same countries, and the same methods.
>
> The point need not be laboured. The experienced administrators will appreciate the need of drawing up a program for a period of years, rather than from year to year, if the development of the Health organisation is to be rational and intelligent.[92]

Along the following years, the joint program was a result of a hard process of discussion and negotiation, in which the League decided the content of the public health programs accordingly to the collaborative orientation and ideology established by the RF, considering that its funding contribution was essential. Nevertheless, the RF did not propose previously its own ideas about the international programs of the League, but it criticized, accepted or disputed their opportunity. After the first period of collaboration, the following grants and programs were approved:

	Expenditures ($)					Appropriations ($) Pledges ($)			
	1922	1923	1924	1925	1926	1927	1928	1929–34	TOT
Interchange Public Health Personnel	15,020	63,080	91,353	83,775	83,775	66,224	50,000		442,937.80
Training Health Statistics		6,645	20,700	19,894	20,580	21,000			
Epidemiological Intelligence Service		29,215	32,808	32,532	32,582	32,840	60,335	218,975	535,047.98
Centre Public Health Documentation						6,937			
Singapore Bureau				26,802	25,000	25,000	20,000	15,000	111,802.27
Conference in Singapore			3,451.09						3,451.09
Expenses Welch-Subcommittee									
Health Committee League			3,087.38						3,087.38
TOTAL	15,020	98,940	151,400	163,004	151,647	152,002	130,335	233,975	1,096,326

Table 1.7: **Expenditures by the League of Nations under Rockefeller Foundation Appropriations to 1926. Appropriations for 1927 and 1928 and pledges for the period 1929–34. Source: G. K. Strode, *Memorandum on The Health Organization of the League of Nations and the Relationship thereto of the International Health Division of the Rockefeller Foundation*, Rockefeller Archive Centre, NY.**

The important amount of $1,096,326 was approved for the interchange of public health experts, the implementation of the Epidemiological Intelligence Service and the international health statistics project, including the consolidation of the Singapore Bureau and a Centre of Documentation in Public Health. The program proposed by Rajchman was well conceived, with good chances of success and logical as a further development of the previous work.

After the first decade of work in international health, the League's activities consisted of certain permanent programs and others temporary depending on special conditions and needs. The permanent ones were the Epidemiological Intelligence Service and the development of an international program of vital statistics and public health documentation, as well as the Standardization programs for biological products, laboratory tests, nutrition and diet and classification of causes of death. The temporary or special ones were devoted to the interchange of public health experts, the creation of technical committees and the celebration of conferences on nutrition, rural health, malaria and trachoma.

Accordingly to these activities, the Rockefeller Foundation agreed on a diminishing scale in aiding routine activities, considering that the 1,000,000 SF contributed by the League were sufficient to keep them at work. The internal debate inside the leading board of the RF was focused upon the support to temporary or special actions considering that the IHD contributed 25 per cent of the total budget. Considering the League's financial situation, Strode believed that during the first half of the 1930s it was unlikely that the League could provide more than 1,000,000 SF per year.[93] In that case, the contribution of the IHD being 25 per cent would represent a total amount under 1,350,000 SF. He calculated that to keep the work of the Health Organization on the 1928 basis, the IHD would have to contribute about 40 per cent of its total budget, which was considered to be too high of a percentage. In addition, there was an objection on the part of the IHD to providing grants to temporary projects: most of them to assist governments in the establishment of permanent bureaux or divisions in their departments of health and these policies were out of the IHD policy when dealing with national governments.

Another objection raised by the RF leaders was mostly political: if the IHD accepted some and rejected other activities, the RF could be accused of directly influencing the Health Organization's policy creating an awkward situation. The IHD considered that the only solution was creating a *Bureau of Studies* in the Health Organization dealing with temporary projects, and in the same manner a *Bureau for Liaison with National Health Administrations* could be set up to take care for international courses of advanced training in public health, interchanges and individual missions.

Being thoroughly convinced as to the importance of the Health Organization in the interwar years, and that its field of activities should not be restricted at the difficult situation created in the early 1930s by the worldwide recession, Strode suggested the following policy and submitted it for the consideration and approval of the IHD:

1 That the permanent and routine activities which are now being aided on the sliding scale principle be declared as being so thoroughly established as to require no further assistance beyond the existing IHD commitments.
2 That the sliding scale principle be applied only to permanent activities.
3 That the activities designated as temporary and special be declared to require additional assistance.
4 That it be suggested that the Health Organization create a Bureau of Studies and a Bureau for Liaison with National Health Administrations to handle the many activities which individually are temporary or limited in character.
5 That the IHD agree to aid the work of these new bureaux over a five or six year period to such an extent that the total commitment of the IHD will not be over one third of the entire Health Organization's budget.
6 That the IHD declare that, at the end of this period, its aid will cease.
7 That the IHD further declare its hope that such developmental aid will permit the Health Organization to so firmly establish its usefulness through these activities that the League will assume their entire cost.[94]

Previous pages show to what extent the power of the RF over the international public health programs of the League was extraordinarily huge. Strode's arguments convinced the leading group and accordingly with this reasoning the RF allocated the following funds:[95]

	Existing Pledges ($)	**Additional Pledge ($)**	**Total ($)**
1930	94,155	5,845	100,000
1931	89,315	10,685	100,000
1932	34,475	65,525	100,000
1933	29,635	70,365	100,000
1934	22,400	77,600	100,000

Table 1.8: **Rockefeller Foundation Funds for the Health Organization of the League of Nations Joint Program (1930–4). Source: G. K. Strode, *Memorandum on The Health Organization of the League of Nations and the Relationship thereto of the International Health Division of the Rockefeller Foundation*, Rockefeller Archive Centre, NY.**

After a period of discussion and negotiation, the Rockefeller Foundation pledged for a period of five years, until the end of 1934, a yearly sum, which should not exceed $144,795. This sum included previous commitments for the Epidemiological Intelligence Service, International Public Health Statistics, the establishment of a Centre of Public Health Documentation and the Interchange of Public Health Officers. In 1931 the previous obligations for these two purposes were respectively $43,715 and $50,000.[96]

During the process of negotiation between Rajchman and Russell for new agreements they referred the possibility of a further arrangement regarding the international coordination of the programs for the instruction of public health officers.[97] This initiative involved meetings of directors of schools and institutes of public health in different countries. Surveys about public health administration included the existing relations between health insurance companies and public health services; consequently it was essential to explore the way of improving them. In a plurality of manners, health insurances were extending not only in America, but also to all European countries. Rajchman reported in Germany of 1,200,000 births occurring annually; 800,000 infants were born of women either insured in their own names or dependent on insured husbands. In Denmark children of members fall automatically under the benefit of the health insurance system and in countries like Austria, England, Poland, Czechoslovakia and others the whole national campaigns against tuberculosis were based on the active participation of the health insurance organizations. In Italy a law approved by the 1930s provided for compulsory insurance against tuberculosis and in many European countries preventive measures against venereal diseases became complementary to the therapeutic activities of the health insurance organizations. Regulations and guiding principles for collaboration between the public administration and insurance companies had been worked out in Germany, Poland and Czechoslovakia. The negotiations between the Rockefeller Foundation and the League of Nations discussed how the initial experience of the different nations in this domain could be transferred to other European countries. In France a social insurance bill, providing for health and invalidity benefits was about to be enacted in 1928 and Japan initiated the second year of a Health Insurance Act. Therefore, this was an essential issue for collaboration between the RF and the League, aiming to boost national negotiations and agreements in the domain of health care initiatives.

One of the topics, which Ludwik Rajchman considered as important in 1926 was the analysis of the benefits of the German *Krankenkassen* system in relation to public health campaigns. Gunn and other leaders of the Rockefeller Foundation, in their studies in different parts of Europe, had been much impressed with the possibilities of a system such as *Krankenkassen* from the point of view of public health and preventive medicine. It is important to keep in mind that the *Krankenkassen* system was based on private organizations, but subjected very strictly to State regulations and control. In as much it was fairly well off; Selskar Gunn reported his expectations: 'Personally I am very glad indeed that the Health Section of the League of Nations is going to make this study. Dr Boudreau, who, by the way has made good, will probably have the direction of this study, although specialists from different countries will participate'.[98] Undoubtedly the organization of public health, health care and health administration at a national level was a very central issue for the League and the Rockefeller leaders. Indeed, Rajchman, in his program for 1926, was planning a study of budgets of federal health services to bring together information with regard to appropriation made for all kinds of health and health related services and activities. He showed his satisfaction for the initiative considering this subject of the most relevance and well within the proper function of the Health Organization of the League of Nations.[99]

To discuss this topic, the Health Committee of the League of Nations appointed a joint commission composed of representatives of insurance companies and public health administrations under the chairmanship of George Newman for the purpose of a joint study of the relations between social insurance companies and national health agencies.[100] Main topics of debate were maternity and infant welfare, hygiene and health of children at school age, tuberculosis prevention and treatment, venereal diseases and public health education. A comparative study on the incidence of tuberculosis was promoted and the League had received enquiries from England, Germany, Austria, Czechoslovakia, Hungary and Denmark. Since the insurance companies kept considerable records and information regarding morbidity, the League proposed introducing modern methods of collection, tabulation, analysis and compilation of data. According to Rajchman 'a comprehensive survey of morbidity and material available for morbidity studies in various countries in Europe is being completed and an analysis both of the list of causes of sickness in use and of certain of the data themselves is being made by the staff of the Health Section and by invited experts'.[101]

Health statistics were to be the background to identifying health problems and the fundamentals of health policies. Germany served as an example. A Statistical Department had been established at the *Allgemeine Ortskrankenkasse* in Berlin under the supervision of Dr Roesle, statistician of the *Reichsgesundheitsamt*. The Department was managed by medical officers and medical statisticians containing data concerning 750,000 insured patients. The Health organization planned to invite selected statisticians working for the *Krankenkassen* to engage the German Statistical Department in the joint study of certain problems selected for investigation by the experts of the Section. The invitation covered officers from different countries constituting an international group able to prepare reports for the joint commission on health insurance and for the Committee of Expert Statisticians of the Health Organization. However, Rajchman had a deep public health perspective and criticized that the medical staff of the insurance companies were not recruited from amongst health officers and often had neither instruction, nor experience about preventive medicine and public health practices. He believed that it was essential to assist those countries where insurance laws were enacted or under parliamentary consideration with a view to preventing mistakes, which might be difficult to repair after the legislations were approved. The League wanted to place at the disposal of Governments the expert advice of officers fully competent on new developments, recruited as far as possible among those associated with joint studies. Rajchman proposed to the Rockefeller IHD to assist such as a program by making available a grant for a period of seven years, which was the period covered by the existing Agreement in regard of the activities of the Health Section in Geneva for an amount of $40,000 per year.[102]

The second proposed program aimed to coordinate academic activities of national schools of hygiene and institutes of public health – including those in Belgrade, Budapest, Prague, Warsaw, Zagreb and later Madrid (1930) – focused on comparative studies on the standardization of serological tests for the diagnosis of syphilis, oral vaccination against typhoid fever, specific vaccines against scarlet fever, rural health facilities and compared studies on nutrition. The expenses of this program were estimated at $25,000 per year including salaries, travelling expenses and grant laboratory expenses.[103]

In 1933 the visible head of the health programs developed by the League experienced a turn. Rajchman was selected by the Council of the League of Nations to act as its delegate in China for twelve months in connection with the program of technical collaboration between the League and the Government of China. Frank Boudreau, a League of Nations health official in China, was elected new Medical Director of the Health Committee.[104] Immediately after assuming his new responsibilities, Boudreau sent to the Rockefeller Foundation a long memorandum of the work previously done together for more than one decade.[105] The general topic of the report was the assistance of the Rockefeller Foundation as cornerstone to the development of the Health Organization of the League of Nations.

In accordance with the information contributed by Boudreau in his detailed memorandum, the Health Section of the League of Nations Secretariat was sufficiently well organized in the winter of 1921–2. Its staff consisted of a director and his secretary-stenographer, a statistical officer and three clerks. Its budget stood at 200,000 SF, but this was a purely theoretical figure for no one really knew what sums were needed or what amounts would be available. Expenditure was 234,387 SF in 1921 and 328,574 SF in 1922.[106]

During its first years of work general doubt prevailed as to what extent it would be possible to demonstrate to the States Members of the League the utility of international health work, and whether the necessary support would be forthcoming from the national health services. In order to consolidate the initiative, attempts to enlist the moral and financial support of the Rockefeller Foundation began in November 1921, culminating a few months later, as we know, in the ratification by the League and the Rockefeller Foundation of two initial collaborative programmes in respect of the International Epidemiological Intelligence Service and Interchanges of Public Health Officials. Since that time further agreements were signed, and by this means the Foundation continued and strengthened its moral and financial support of the Health Organization.

It is important to keep in mind that in the absence of US active diplomacy, the funds from the RF acquired great political relevance.

During the most critical period in 1921–3, the diplomatic encouragement and financial support of the Rockefeller Foundation was perhaps one of the decisive factors in ensuring the continuity and growth of the new international health organization, which came to play an important part in the general work of stabilization policies of the League. Malnutrition, contagious diseases such as malaria, trachoma or tuberculosis, epidemics and standardization of biological products were not only relevant for health, they also represented main political agents in the post war years.

After a decade, the technical authority of the Health Organization was undisputed, either by policy makers and governments, or by national health authorities. The friends of international collaboration believed that the League had successfully demonstrated the possibility of utilizing public health work for the advancement of international technical collaboration as well as of international understanding on a world basis. The work of the Health Organization, while it was publicly shown as purely technical, had an undisputable political dimension and exercised a considerable influence on the progress of international collaboration through the League in its stabilization policies. The success achieved in health policies enabled the opening of the way for international work in such fields as education, economics and transport, thanks to an efficient implementation of material resources overcoming national prejudices and preventions when facing health policies, usually considered to be internal affairs of national governments. The League's work in China afforded an excellent example. Starting with health policies in 1929, further developments and technical collaborative programmes in education, economics, transport and agriculture were initiated in China. In the early 1930s, the possibilities in this direction were only limited by financial and staff resources.

In 1933 a meaningful change in the personal representation took place. Rajchman was appointed by the Council of the League of Nations to act as delegate in China for a period of twelve months in connection with the program of technical collaboration between the League and the Government of China.[107] Boudreau substituted Rajchman as Medical Director of the Health Organization and immediately retook contacts and negotiations with the Rockefeller Foundation.[108] To start with, he sent a global report of the work done until then by the HO and the role played by the essential assistance of the RF since its inception.

In 1933, the staff of the Health Section consisted of a Medical Director, seventeen technical officers and a series of subordinate personnel numbering thirty-five.[109] Nearly one hundred experts on the staff of Governments, research institutes and laboratories, as well as universities were carrying out work in most of the regions of the world on behalf of the Health Organization of the League. The Service of Epidemiological Intelligence at Geneva and Singapore received information from every organized health administration in the world and transmitted its epidemiological bulletins daily, weekly and monthly by wireless, telegraph and postal services. National Institutes of Medical Research and Experimental Medicine in several countries kept its international standard preparations for biological products, serological preparations and vaccines. Those laboratories tested national standards and sent samples to national laboratories on request. This international laboratory medicine was strongly boosted by the League being the State Serum Institute at Copenhagen and the National Institute for Medical Research at Hampstead the most important repositories of international standards for the Health Organization.

In the context of the several programs, technical representatives of the Health Organization were frequently attached temporarily to Health Administrations in countries such as China, Czechoslovakia, Greece, Hungary and Italy. In China and Greece the National Health Services were being organized according to schemes drawn up on behalf of the Health Organization by public health experts from the leading countries. Work entrusted to the Health Organization by international conferences and by the Assembly and Council of the League of Nation was carried out on its behalf by national health institutes, laboratories and schools of hygiene in ten cities: Copenhagen, Warsaw, Prague, Budapest, Zagreb, Nancy, Madrid, Cambridge, Berlin and Jassy (Romania). With the collaboration of those prominent institutions, courses and practical work on the control of malaria had been organized on behalf of the Health Organization in four of the leading Institutes in Europe (Hamburg, London, Paris and Rome), complemented with practical work in the rural districts of three European countries (Italy, Spain and Yugoslavia), where malaria was prevalent as a social disease and a serious medical problem. These activities were later extended to the East, and malaria courses for the benefit of Eastern malariologists were developed at Singapore in 1934. As we shall comment in more detail in another chapter, to reinforce international health, the French Government agreed to create in Paris an International School of Hygiene placing it at the disposal of the Health Organization of the League of Nations for the benefit of its system of interchanges of officials, coordination of the programs of the national schools of hygiene and individual study tours. It was supposed to become a sort of coordinating body for directors and health authorities. In addition, the Government of Brazil decided to set aside funds for the establishment of an anti-leprosy centre at Rio de Janeiro in 1934, under the auspices of the League.

Since the Rockefeller Foundation first made a grant to the Health Organization for the interchange of public health personnel on an international scale in 1922 until 1934, thirty-five collective study tours had been organized, which involved visits to thirty-one countries by 587 health officers who came from more than sixty countries.[110] In addition, individual missions had been granted to 175 health officers from thirty-eight countries, and 105 malariologists had participated in the international malaria courses. This program was probably the one, which involved more clearly an international perspective with the aim at creating an international elite of experts in public health, constituting a perfectly connected network, sharing instructive programs, a similar public health ideology and showing world-wide capacity of action. The interchange program received, from the beginning, substantial material support and technical advice from the League.

This brief review of the Health Organization's activities sent by Boudreau to Strode served to show that the technical authority of the HO was unchallenged and its influence and capacity of intervention increased worldwide. Indeed, from 1921 to 1930 the Health Organization's growth was constant and rapid due to the permanent increase of international demands on public health. As a consequence, the sums set aside for the HO in the general budget of the League increased as well. In 1926 the budget was stabilized at one million gold francs, and this amount was maintained until 1930. Stabilization was imposed on the Health Organization to preserve a due proportion between its development and that of the other technical organs of the League. In 1931 they amounted to more than 1,300,000 SF, to which should be added another 120,000 SF for work in Latin America. In 1932 and subsequent years, the League's budgets also included an item for technical assistance to China to defray, among other things, the cost of certain health enquiries in that country. In 1933, for example, 15,000 SF were set aside for health work in China under this item. In addition some $36,000 (normally equivalent to 104,400 SF) contributed to Far Eastern Governments towards the support of the Singapore Bureau.[111]

These sums were included for the Health Organization by the Assembly of the League of Nations in accordance with the governments involved. However the world economic depression had negative effects on the budget of the League at that time. Boudreau considered that otherwise it would have been fairly easy to increase the amounts contributed by the State members towards the Health Organization so as to provide in 1935 for taking over and maintaining the work hitherto supported by the IHD of the Rockefeller Foundation. Nevertheless, the bad economic situation in which many of the State members of the League found themselves during the 1930s made it difficult for them to obtain the necessary amounts of foreign currency with which to pay their contributions. Therefore, the amount of contributions received by the League dropped considerably, representatives of the Governments cried for economy and the Assembly was forced to reduce budgets and expenditure. The Health Organization budget for 1934 was expected to be 900,000 SF including some 80,000 SF for technical work in Latin America, and it was expected that the contributions of Far Eastern Governments to the Singapore Bureau would amount to $31,556. The conclusion drawn by Boudreau was overwhelming: if the Health Organization could not count 'on the generous grant of the Rockefeller Foundation' in 1934, it would have to cope with a very difficult situation.

Under those hard circumstances the situation was irreversible and the HO depended absolutely on the grants and the will of the Rockefeller leaders. Obviously they showed sensibility and the second agreement with the Rockefeller Foundation came to an end by 31 December 1934. The Health Organization could hardly count on receiving from the League in 1935 more than one million SF, plus seventy or eighty thousand SF for work in Latin-America and $20,000 to $30,000 for the Singapore Bureau a sum notably insufficient for program continuity, but a sort of oxygen tank for its hard survival.

Indeed should further support from the Rockefeller Foundation not be forthcoming the immediate negative effects on the Health Organization would be under very critical circumstances. Clearly negotiation happened under enormous pressure, a pressure used by the League authorities to put the RF against the wall, but at the same time giving the American foundation a huge capacity of decision. So far, in spite of the reduction in its budget, due to lessening contributions from the states members and the reduced gold value of its Rockefeller Grant, the HO leaders boasted about having been capable to maintain its high standard and consolidate the programs by measures of rationalization and sound administration. Notwithstanding the situation expected for 1935, and subsequent years, was to be much more difficult. Practically all members of its technical staff previously paid from the Rockefeller Foundation grants would have to be dismissed. In practical terms that implied fifteen out of a total of forty-two posts would be vacated, among them those of the two most senior medical officers in the Health Organization.[112] Of the eighteen medical officers on the staff of the Health Section, ten would have to leave; the sums set aside for interchanges and individual missions would be reduced by 68 per cent, and the credits for printing the international epidemiological records were practically unfeasible.[113]

In addition, if the predictions were true it would be very difficult to maintain the activities of the Singapore Bureau at more than the lowest level, and the already reduced credits for the general technical work of the Section such as the biological standards research, the malaria investigation and campaigns, the fight against opium, the international agreements and research on nutrition, as well as the programs to discuss rural hygiene, among others, would be diminished to such a level that only 'routine performance of tasks laid upon the Health Organization by international agreements could be carried out'.[114] Much of the League's assistance to Governments, which had appealed to it in increasing numbers in previous years would have to give up, either in connection with schemes calling for the organization of health services or in special fields such as the control of malaria. The final consequence was ominous for international health: the Health Organization would have to relinquish the leadership, which had enabled its initiatives to pave the way for international technical collaboration in several sanitary fields. Particularly, the work encouraged by the League to bring about an improved esprit of collaboration between national health services and policy makers, stimulating collaborative networks and international expert commissions, all these initiatives could be seriously reduced, if not entirely stopped. Boudreau was compelling in his conclusion:

> While it was probable that the Assembly would seek to prevent this maximum reduction in the activities of the Health Organisation, which would weaken the strength and influence of the League as a whole, no one conversant, with the political and economic situation at that time, could cope that more than a modicum of success would crown the efforts of those Governments which might seek to obtain from the League the vote of sums sufficient to make up for the withdrawal of support on the part of the Rockefeller Foundation.[115]

The official position of the League differed from that of particular Governments in a variety of ways. In the first place the HO was a new institution working in the relatively new field of international health. Duration was the most important element in the effort to consolidate its position and from this point of view the Health Organization was very young as such institutions go. The rhythm of its development could not be the same as that of governmental institutions; in international matters development naturally took place at a much slower speed. It was generally understood that during a comparatively long period the machinery of the League was not really utilized for major political and economic operations in the international field. However, it was only during the 1930s that the severe tests to which it was to be subjected in future would let know to what extent it was utilized by the governments of many countries as the most important instrument in the regulation of international affairs. In consequence, if it was not to perish, the strength of its component parts had to be maintained and even improved. Many authorities believed that the HO was one of the important parts of the international health machinery, because of the comparative ease with which international collaboration in health matters had been established and the appeal to expertise, which it had made to large groups in every country.[116]

There were probably many other reasons why the League should not have the same conditions applied to it, which were imposed on Governments receiving grants from the Rockefeller Foundation. Among others, its officers could not make the same pledges as the officials of individual Governments; their action was subject to more rigid control by a larger number of official bodies with different aims and standards. In the case of the League when regarding health matters, it was argued that future action should be predicated upon past experience. Prior to the worldwide economic depression affecting the 1930s, the substantial yearly increases in the budget of the HO were a proof that League officials were doing everything in their power to consolidate its position so as to enable it to take over the activities supported by the Rockefeller Foundation.

Significantly Boudreau showed a very pessimistic assessment of the situation, considering the widespread of nationalism and assuming the difficulties derived from the serious economic situation. Therefore, the League had come to another turning of the road, and its Health Organization suffered from the second crisis in its development. Under those circumstances, the main question was how to secure that the withdrawal of the Rockefeller grant affected not so seriously all HO programs and, to some extent, the League itself, as to reduce the role of the former to such a degree that it will no longer be an important factor in the development of the previous scheme of health policies based on international technical collaboration. In fact, under such difficult circumstances, further assistance from the Rockefeller Foundation towards the fundamental activities of the HO, previously supported up to the mid-1930s, was considered to be the only material possibility to survive.[117] The future of the HO was in the hands of the Rockefeller Foundation.

In order to avoid the dismissal of officials traditionally paid from the Rockefeller chapter of the budget, and therefore weakening seriously the structure and dimension of the staff, Boudreau believed that 'it would be necessary to maintain the grant of the RF in 1935 at the present figure, that is $144,795, for with the dollar at its present exchange rate, the value of the grant has also decreased considerably'.[118] Those were difficult times. In subsequent years it was only natural that the grant should be somewhat reduced in view of the general economic depression, which had forced all Governments to apply severe cuts in order to rationalize expenses. But the leaders of the HO made an effort to be optimistic considering that the social and economic crisis would improve gradually, so that such a method would enable the League to take over the support of projects assisted by the Rockefeller Foundation. The League officials concerned made efforts to show that they had the will to work towards this end and they probably were sincere, but the development of events would prove them wrong.

As a result of the proposed reduction in the grant of the Rockefeller Foundation after 1935 would be the gradual adjustment of the HO to enable its main programs and activities to be carried out at a more restrictive cost. The main target was to make such an adjustment without doing serious harm to the core aspects of the activities, providing it could be done gradually and methodically. As a strategy in this direction, during the previous years an increasing percentage of the work formerly carried out at Geneva had been shifted to experts, national health officers in the employ of Governments, scientific institutions and universities. This strategy would have been impossible in the beginning, when confidence in the usefulness of the HO activities had not been fully established. This decentralization of a part of the activities enabled the Section to place five of its medical officers in important health positions in their own respective countries, where they were paid by the Government. But this policy had a limit beyond which the reduction in the central work and staff of the section could not go without danger of permanent harm resulting. A nucleus of first class technical officers, experienced in international health work and on the permanent staff of the League was absolutely necessary. One of the greatest benefits conferred on the HO by the support of the Rockefeller Foundation was the opportunity to employ and maintain a highly specialized technical staff, without those restrictions as to nationality and salary, which should be safeguarded in regular League appointments.

Just before the Boudreau memorandum, the League Assembly held in Geneva in November 1933 ended under a critical landscape shadowed by serious disarmament difficulties. Many national delegates spoke about the necessity of restricting the non-essential work of the League to permit the concentration of all effort on the prevention of war, but practically all who spoke in those terms, made it perfectly clear that the work of the Health Organization was essential and did not have to be unduly restricted.

In July 1933 the French diplomat Joseph Avenol was appointed second Secretary-General of the League of Nations. Just a few months later, on 5 December 1933, Strode was invited to a private dinner, in which Avenol expressed the League's desire to continue with the RF Joint Program. Avenol assessed the importance of the RF for the HO programs and explained to Strode the immediate plans in international health. The Assembly planned to provide the HO with around 1,000,000 SF in 1934 considering the importance of its work, keeping a certain sense of proportion between the various technical organizations, which in practical terms meant that any increase in the budget of one could not be done without proportional increases in the others. Obviously, under the present circumstances the League was not ready to gradually take over the RF grants.[119] The perspective of the RF was, however, substantially different, inasmuch as the aims which the RF had in view when it became initially interested and engaged in the work of the HO, it seemed to have attained. The RF thought that it might be doing a disservice to the Health Organization in helping to maintain the collaboration at a financial level, which could not be supported when the RF withdrew. Strode summarized the state of the budgets in his report to the Rockefeller authorities:[120]

Year	Estimated Expenditure LNHO (SF)	Grants RF (SF)
1932	1,735,498	750,414
1933	1,633,665	652,663
1934	1,364,000	464,000

Table 1.9: **Estimated Expediture of the Rockefeller Foundation Funds for the Health Organization of the League of Nations Joint Program (1932–4). Source: Letter No. 387 from G.K. Strode to F.F. Russell (1933). Rockefeller Archive Centre, NY.**

These numbers indicate that the calculated decrease of the HO expenditure during the three years period of 1932–4 was 22 per cent and the decrease of the RF grant was 38 per cent. Negotiations and budgets show a deep crisis in the HO during the first years of the 1930s, although it was generally recognized that the work of the Health Organization, while purely technical, had exercised a considerable influence on the progress of international collaboration. During the previous years, the League had been able to open the way for international work in such fields as education, economics and transport thanks to its material resources and the comparative absence of vested interests and national prejudices in health matters. The League's work in China was an excellent example of success. Starting with health as soon as 1929, China sought and obtained the technical collaboration of the League in education, economics, transport, agriculture and other matters. After the first impulse, going forward to improve this direction was something only limited by the lack of resources in professional, well-trained staff and financial funds.

As a matter of fact, the bad economic situation in which many of the State members of the League found themselves in 1931, 1932 and 1933 made it difficult for them to obtain the necessary amounts of foreign currency with which to pay their contributions to the League. Therefore, the amount of national contributions dropped considerably, representatives of most Governments claimed for economy and the Assembly was forced to reduce budgets and expenditure. The Health Organization budget for 1934 was finally fixed at 900,000 SF. Moreover some 80,000 SF were allocated for technical work in Latin-America, and it was expected that the contributions of Far Eastern Governments to the Singapore Bureau will amount to $31,556. In the process of negotiation, the main argument was that if the Health Organization could not count, in 1934, on the generous grant of the Rockefeller Foundation, it would be in an unbearable situation. The representatives of the League highlighted that under the critical economic circumstances the Health Organization could hardly count on receiving from the League in 1935 more than one million SF, plus seventy or eighty thousand for work in Latin America and $20,000 to $30,000 dollars for the Singapore Bureau.

In short, before the signature of a new agreement, the threat of a big financial crisis for the Health Organization was serious. If further support from the Rockefeller Foundation were not forthcoming, the continuity of the programs would be seriously affected. So far, in spite of the reduction in its budget due to lessening contributions from the States Members and the reduced gold value of the Rockefeller Grant, the HO had been capable to maintain efficiency and consolidate programs by adjustment measures. But the expectations for 1935 and subsequent years were much more difficult. The HO was strongly dependent upon the grant of the Rockefeller Foundation for its continuity.

Another unavoidable effect would be giving up much of the assistance offered to Governments, which had requested it in increasing numbers in previous years, either in connection with schemes calling for the complete reorganization of their health services or in special fields such as the control of malaria. The Health Organization would have to relinquish that leadership which had enabled it to pave the way for the promotion of international health and the coordination of technical collaboration in specific fields. It was not a matter of political decision by the Assembly in favour of the continuity of the HO, something that was already consolidated at that time. Continuity depended upon enough money. The Assembly tried to prevent the extreme reduction in the activities of the HO, which would weaken the strength and the influence of the League as a whole, but no one aware of the critical political and economic situation could imagine the League would crown the efforts of the Governments which might seek to obtain from the League the amount of grants sufficient to make up for the withdrawal of support on the part of the Rockefeller Foundation.

Starting the second half of 1936, Strode sent the semi-annual report of the Paris Office of the Rockefeller Foundation to the central office in New York. He informed them that the twenty-third session of the Health Committee was convened 29 April 1936. This was the last meeting the present committee could hold since its three-year mandate terminated in 1936.[121] The Secretariat was charged with drafting a plan for reorganization of the Committee and negotiations respecting this were under way with the *Office International d'Hygiène Publique* in Paris. So far, no plan had been evolved but some arrangements had to be made before the end of the year in such a critical moment. The Bureau, enjoying certain executive functions and responsibilities, would hold its June meeting in Moscow as a guest of the Russian government.

The work of the Health Organization did not need be reviewed in detail at this time since there had been no significant changes from what was reported at the end of 1935. The major interests continued to focus on the two main programs of the improvement of nutrition and housing. Committees set up to handle these programs had been active and considerable progress had been made. The third topic, physical education, which with nutrition and housing became the centre of interest during the early thirties, was later on getting started as an international cooperative study. The Health Section prepared a preliminary report, which was intended to serve as a basis for further development and implementation of the subject.

The last of the financial grants in support of the Health Organization, made by the IHD of the RF, was to terminate at the end of 1937. For the first time, therefore, the Health Organization would be faced with the necessity of operating within the budgetary limits provided by the League itself. According with the traditional Rockefeller collaborative ideology, there was reason to believe that this necessity would have a positive effect and was greatly to be desired. The funds provided for 1937 from League sources approached some 800,000 SF, which together with 300,000 SF assured by the Rockefeller IHD grant gave a global budget of 1,100,000 SF. As a matter of fact, the League became immersed in a delicate situation at the end of the 1930s. To compensate for the IHD grant, that would no longer be available in 1938, the Health Section was forced to persuade the League to raise its contribution to 1,100,000 SF for that year, but there was no assurance that it would be done and the international situation turned more and more complicated.[122]

2 THE FIRST GREAT INTERVENTION: EPIDEMICS AND FAMINE IN EASTERN EUROPE

The first international coordinated effort to fight epidemics in Europe on the part of governmental public health services was boosted in March 1920 by the Council of the League of Nations. An international sanitary conference was convened in London in close cooperation with the representatives of the Polish Public Health Service to submit a plan for a campaign against the serious outbreak of typhus in wide regions of Poland. The conference launched successive appeals for funds to all Governments participating in the meeting, and an Epidemic Commission was appointed to administer the funds and to be instrumental in bringing material assistance to the public health services concerned.[1] During January 1922, information had accumulated at the Health Section showing that the situation in Eastern Europe was rapidly impaired and becoming more serious, both in regards to the extension of the famine in Russia and the greatly increased incidence of epidemic diseases, with a resulting temporary breakdown of the sanitary defences in the Eastern provinces of Poland. The Secretariat of the League of Nations consequently circulated a report on the health situation in Eastern Europe to all States Members of the League to prompt an awareness of the dimension of the health problem as a risk factor for political instability during the sensible post-war years.

Epidemiological records available showed that since 1914 cholera had, in rural districts of Russia, yearly epidemic outbreaks, which became increasingly serious after the Bolshevik revolution and the Great War. The numbers were:[2]

Year	Cholera Cases	Year	Cholera Cases
1914	9,715	1915	66,455
1916	1,800	1917	130
1918	41,586	1919	5,119
1920	29,615	1921	207,389
1922	86,178		

Table 2.1: ***Dr Syssin's Report to the League of Nations.*** **Rockefeller Archive Centre, NY.**

The situation had become so extreme by the early 1920s that the international health experts urged measures and the London Conference recommended setting up an Epidemic Commission to coordinate the efforts to deal with the expansion of the epidemics mainly in Russia, Poland and the Baltic States. The Commission assisted the national authorities by means of public health experts, medicines, sanitary equipment and food supply, among other materials. In addition the implementation of preventive measures and the establishment of sanitary cordons became necessary as a consequence of the war between Poland and Russia. Hundreds of thousands of refugees returned to Poland and the Baltic States after the war from Siberia and other areas of Central Russia. Out of any control, the situation was hard to manage requiring preventive measures, safe and efficient transport and organized systems for the relief and settlement of the crowds of refugees.

The agreement between the Health Section of the League and the Russian sanitary authorities represented by the Health Minister Dr Siemashko, was at the time the only diplomatic link between the League of Nations and the Russian Government. In addition, under existing conditions of shortage of physicians, much of the epidemiological information was gathered and transmitted by *feldshers*[3] and other non-professional staff acting as primary health care agents in rural areas. Therefore supplementary efforts to improve the reliability of the official records had to be applied to confirm diagnosis when diseases such as cholera, smallpox, typhus and other contagious diseases were reported without either laboratory tests or clinical expertise in Western medicine. In this direction, the League expert members of the Epidemic Commission worked in cooperation with the Russian authorities, but in some aspects the relationship was not easy.[4]

When the Epidemic Commission of the League started its cooperation with Russian authorities there were in the country tweny-five official health laboratories. The international experts were informed about their facilities, not fully equipped but most of them had basic equipment of apparatus, autoclaves etc.[5] The international commission made a report to improve their efficiency considering that the greatest need of the Russian laboratories was an annual budget for smaller instruments and simple facilities, and laboratory materials for routine research and better salaries, which involved instruction and recognition for the laboratory experts. The Epidemic Commission recommended the League to provide the Russian health authorities a grant to improve those laboratory facilities as well as to solve the serious need of a school of hygiene, preferably situated in Moscow, organized like the national school of hygiene in Warsaw and other European cities.

In spite of the political tensions and distrust, the experts of the Epidemic Commission believed that the Russian Government wanted cooperation in such a way that the international experts and financial aid could contribute to the improvement of the control of infectious diseases. The documents kept in the League of Nations Archives and in the Rockefeller Archive Centre show that the relationship between international experts and Russian officers was courteous and cooperative and the League received the best reports of Russian professors of the Health Department at Moscow, Kharkov and Rostov.[6]

Nevertheless, the Epidemic Commission was not conceived as a charitable relief organization. Its funds were derived from subscriptions contributed by Governments, who recognized that the extermination of typhus in Eastern Europe was not a regional problem but a matter of international concern. It did not undertake independent work, but it acted through the public health administration of the countries concerned. Strengthening the health organization of the nations was considered to be the most effective means to cope with the spread of epidemics. It differed fundamentally from the ordinary relief organizations interested in the immediate alleviation of suffering of the affected population or in satisfying the immediate needs under catastrophic situations, with the result that, when assistance was withdrawn, former conditions again prevailed. The Epidemic Commission acted on the principle that a permanent system of sanitary defence should be built up in Eastern Europe on the border zone forming the bridge between Poland and Russia.[7]

Created under exceptional circumstances, the Epidemic Commission was the only health agency of the League until September 1921, when, after very prolonged negotiations, the Second Assembly set up the Health Organization with the Health Section of the Permanent Secretariat as its executive organ. The Epidemic Commission became an active part of the Health Organization, since the latter decided immediately to obtain accurate information concerning the epidemiological situation and the health conditions of the most affected areas in Europe. The good political relations with Poland, Czechoslovakia and the Baltic States did not suffice for that purpose, and a special Commission was dispatched to Moscow in order to establish contacts with the Russian People's Health Commissariat, the administrative agency in charge of health politics. This diplomatic approach facilitated the presence of representatives of the Epidemic Commission in Russia, and therefore more accurate epidemiologic information from both Russia and Ukraine was received regularly. All reports were presented to the Warsaw Conference (1922), playing an important role in the assessment of the real dimension of the problem.

The Polish Government received the experts' report and, therefore, applied to the Council's President of the League, requesting the immediate convocation of a technical European Conference to consider the situation and the measures to be taken to prevent the further spread of the disease, as well as the necessity of attacking it at the central sites of the epidemics. The Conference, in full agreement and coordination with the League of Red Cross Societies and the Committee of the *Office International d'Hygiène Publique*, declared that the epidemic situation in Eastern Europe was so menacing for the entire continent; entailing such heavy burdens on the states concerned that the task of fighting epidemics was beyond the capacity of national administrations involved and voluntary associations. The Conference, therefore, urged that this task be entrusted to the only official international organization with sufficient authority and power to undertake and coordinate the work, namely, the League of Nations.

The Epidemic Commission was appointed, headed by Norman White, a British Public Health Officer with long anti-epidemic experience in India. The Commission received complete autonomy of work, but was responsible to the Council for its activities and was specifically appointed for the purpose of fighting epidemics in Eastern Europe. For both epidemiological and financial reasons, the Commission began its work in Poland. Since the funds placed at its disposal by the governments members of the League – some £136,000 – were not large enough to make possible an anti-epidemic campaign on the scale originally planned, the Commission confined itself to delivering to the Polish health authorities a series of essential aspects related to the technical organization in the fight against epidemics, such as the organization of motor transport, availability of soap, hygienic clothing and some medical facilities most needed at the outset of the campaign, as well as providing funds for the repair and equipment of bathing and disinfecting establishments, quarantine stations, hospitals and other public spaces. The Commission also delivered fifty complete bed hospital units.[8]

The work initiated by the Epidemic Commission in cooperation with the Polish health authorities was a first experiment in international sanitary cooperation on a large scale and, after a first evaluation, it was considered to have been a conspicuous success.[9] But as the epidemic situation in Russia became greatly aggravated in the autumn of 1921, it represented a serious menace to its Western neighbours, owing to the influence of famine and malnutrition in impairing the state of health of the population and stimulating uncontrolled mass migrations. Therefore, it was felt that more drastic and far-reaching measures were necessary to cope with the resulting situation and avoid uncontrolled expansion.

Finally the Conference was accordingly held in Warsaw, from 20–8 March, 1922, and consisted of twenty-seven nations, namely Austria, Belgium, Bulgaria Czechoslovakia, Denmark, Esthonia, Finland, France, Germany, Great Britain, Greece, Holland, Hungary, Italy, Japan, Latvia, Lithuania, Norway, Poland, Rumania, Serb-Croat-Slovene State, Soviet Russia, Soviet Ukraine, Spain, Sweden, Switzerland and Turkey. The Free City of Danzig was also represented.[10]

From the constitutional point of view this conference was of considerable interest, since it was convened by Poland as a member of the League of Nations with the approval of the Council, and in reliance on the help of the League Organizations. Germany, Soviet Russia, Soviet Ukraine, Hungary and Turkey, all of them non-members of the League, were represented at the conference, being the first general European conference in which Soviet Russia and Soviet Ukraine had ever taken part.[11] The democratic and truly international character of the conference is also significant, each delegation having one vote and decisions being passed by a majority, something certainly hard in a time of conflicts and high international tensions. According to the chronicle, German language was in practice more generally used than either of the official languages: English and French. The Conference was thus an all-European and a semi-League affair, and represented a tribute to the elasticity and adaptability of the League's machinery, a test of its ability to intervene in international affairs and an expression of the 'potential universality of the League itself'.[12]

It was decided to break up into three Committees and the Bureau of the Conference was constituted as follows:

- Dr Chodzko (Poland), President.
- Dr Terburgh (the Netherlands), Vice-president.
- Dr Cruveilhier (France), Vice-president.
- Dr Groenlund (Finland), Vice-president.
- Colonel James (Great Britain), President of the First Committee.
- Dr Frey (Germany), President of the Second Committee.
- Dr Messea (Italy), President of the Third Committee.
- Prof. Cantacuzene (Romania), Vice-president of the First Committee.
- Dr Kulhavy (Czechoslovakia), Vice-president of the First Committee.
- Dr Stampar (Serb-Croat-Slovene State), Vice-president of the Second Committee.
- Dr Van Boegkel (Belgium), Vice-president of the Second Committee.
- Dr Kalina (Russia), Vice-president of the Third Committee.
- Dr Naeslund (Sweden), Vice-president of the Third Committee.

The First Committee assessed the epidemiological situation on the basis of the very detailed reports presented by Estonia, Latvia, Lithuania, Poland, Romania, Russia, Turkey and the Ukraine. Colonel James acted as rapporteur of this committee. The Second Committee discussed the measures to be taken by countries adjoining Russia and by neighbouring States to ensure the exchange of information concerning the evolution of the epidemics and to reach agreement as to the means for preventing the further spread of the epidemics from a regional and international perspective. Dr Kolinsky acted as rapporteur.

The Third Committee was entrusted with the preparation of a detailed program of sanitary defence in the frontier zone between the border-states and Russia and the Ukraine, as well as to propose measures of direct fight against the epidemics at their centres of origin.

In view of the complex magnitude of the work of this Committee, the President, with the consent of the Bureau, appointed a Sub-Committee, under the chairmanship of Dr Maxa (Czechoslovakia), to consider in detail the program brought forward in each case by the national delegations. Professor Otto (Germany), Professor Maggiora (Italy), Dr Haigh, Dr Syssin and Dr Kalina (Russia) and Dr Kholodny (Ukraine) examined the Russian and Ukrainian program to cope with the epidemiological emergency. Professor Cantacuzene (Roumania) and Colonel Gauthier examined the Polish Program; Professor Otto and Dr Mutermilch reported on the Lithuanian program; Dr Sztolcman (Poland) reported the Lett and Estonian programs, while Professor Cantacuzene placed before the Committee a plan of future action for Romania.[13] Minutes express with detail the huge amount of information made available to the Conference.

The guidelines and strategies proposed by the various Sub-Committees were discussed by experts participating in the conference as mentioned above with the help of Colonel James (Great Britain) and Professor Castellani (Italy). The First Committee considered the report presented by the Health Section of the League of Nations, the Russian, Polish, Czecho-Slovak, Estonian, Lithuanian, Latvian and Romanian Delegates' reports, as well as a series of reports presented by Dr Haigh, who was able to lay before the Committee the results of his tour of inspection in Russia and the Ukraine.[14] Professor Muehlens, who worked in Russia as Head of the German Red Cross Mission at Moscow and had a long experience in the famine areas, also furnished the Committee with very full information on the epidemic situation in the interior of Russia. The Romanian and Polish Delegates presented as well detailed information on the progress of epidemic diseases in their countries.

Before the end of the Conference Ludwik Rajchman, on the invitation of the President, summarized the results achieved.[15] He reminded the delegates that on the 22 March the Plenary Meeting had passed a general resolution based on the reports presented by members of the Health Section of the League and by the national delegations of Poland, Russia, Ukraine, Estonia, Latvia and Lithuania. Rajchman said that the Conference had analyzed these reports in detail and listened to remarkable statements made by Professor Muehlens (Germany) and Dr Haigh, as a representative of the Health Section of the League, before the First and the Third Committees. They acted as impartial eyewitnesses trying to contribute illustrations of the general epidemiological conditions in Russia.

As a result of the information circulated and the discussion, the Conference had resolved to place on record that the epidemic situation in Eastern Europe had reached its most critical stage by 1920, and that thanks to the efforts of the Public Health Services of the countries involved, the first nine months of 1921 had shown a very marked improvement in the epidemiological situation. However the famine and the consequent movements of population had created, by November, a sudden increase in all the epidemics. Cholera had appeared again in the Ukraine in December, and, thereafter, it was continuing to spread westwards in an alarming manner. The Conference had very rightly pointed out serious danger and the necessity of taking immediate action at an international level.

The first immediate measure to be taken was that of defence, trying to stop the scope and preventing the further spread of the epidemics.

The Second Committee had examined the question of how far the provisions settled at the Paris Convention of 1912 were applicable to both modern notions of etiology and epidemiology and to the extraordinary impairment of the present health conditions in Eastern Europe. They had decided that the main principles of the Paris Convention should be adhered to, but they had suggested a number of modifications to be introduced in any agreements negotiated between individual States. Those modifications had been laid down in a series of statements, which it was hoped might guide the negotiating governments.

The conference established a good cooperative atmosphere and all the Delegations present at the Conference agreed to exchange full information of the health conditions in their respective countries. Only this commitment represented a great advance for international health diplomacy. However Rajchman considered that the Delegations to the Conference had done more than this. Wishing to emphasize their anxiety to start immediate practical collaborative work, the delegates had expressed their willingness to start negotiations at once. The Polish and Czechoslovakian delegates had opened negotiations about the epidemiologic problems affecting the situation in both countries on the previous day. The Latvian and the Polish, the Romanian and the Polish Governments started negotiations as well immediately after the Conference. And Rajchman was convinced that the Russian Delegation was ready to open without delay conversations with Latvia, Estonia and Finland regarding the state of the sanitary conventions, in full agreement with the Delegations of those countries. He felt authorized to state that the Czechoslovakian Delegation was prepared to open negotiations with the German Delegation and that Poland was equally ready to begin conversations with the German Delegation. He had been asked by both parties to say that the negotiations between Poland and the Russian and Ukrainian Delegations had only been interrupted temporarily owing to the additional work of the Warsaw Conference. In short, the hard epidemic outbreak in Eastern Europe in the early 1920s opened the doors to a wide diplomatic activity put into action by the sanitary authorities of most European countries and the Health Organization of the League of Nations was the backbone. The great international reaction was a strong push to consolidate the importance of health diplomacy inside the League of Nations.[16]

The Conference unanimously resolved that means should be provided for mediation in case of differences arising as to the interpretation and application of these conventions, and had recommended that this work should be entrusted to the Health Organization of the League as a neutral and technical body. The Conference not only analyzed the epidemic situation and the hazards derived from it; measures to prevent the further spread of these diseases were also suggested, studying the most difficult problem of attacking the epidemics at their source. The Third

Committee did the technical analysis of the situation and several sub-committees studied in detail the proposals brought forward by a number of national delegations. Up to the Warsaw Conference this problem had always been discussed from the point of view of the defence of the rest of Europe against the danger of epidemics spreading from their usual centres in Eastern Europe or in the colonies.

All European countries agreed to take an active part in the campaign against the epidemics. The allocation of expenses in the case of States Members active at the League of Nations were to be made in accordance with the scale adopted by the Second Assembly. All other participating States were asked to contribute their share of the expenses on a similar basis, while States conducting the campaign in their country at their own expenses were allowed to deduct the expenditure from their quota. Contributions could be made in money, supplies or personnel.[17]

A convincing conclusion was apparent to everybody: that no scheme of economic reconstruction of the Eastern European countries, and consequently of the whole of Europe, was possible until effective measures against the epidemics had been taken and the critical situation overcome. The delegates had decided to impress upon their respective governments the only possible view, that the problem of the economic and social recovery of Europe affected every European nation not only the more damaged, and that consequently every European State was necessarily interested and should feel itself committed in remedying the epidemic hazard.

The Third Committee had examined very carefully the state of sanitary defence both in Russia and the Ukraine and also in the countries bordering on those States. Each national report had been analyzed by a small sub-committee, consisting of experts whose authority was recognized. Members of the respective national delegations had given full statements of their needs, and of their strong and their weak points. The expression *sanitary defence* was made to apply to the defence of the Eastern frontiers of Poland, Rumania, Latvia and Estonia, against the epidemics spread from Russian regions. The Conference extended its reach to include Russia itself despite the difficult relations with the Soviet government. The experts were convincing on the fact that vital parts of Russian territory should be guarded as well against the hazard of infections coming from epidemic areas and that special attention should be paid to health measures on the railway and waterway communications as the most important lines along which the diseases spread.[18]

The Italian and the German Delegations had insisted upon the importance of doing away with the expressions *sanitary cordon* and *quarantine*. They had reasonably pointed out that quarantine was never complete scientifically speaking unless accompanied by bacteriological examinations, a procedure impracticable in the countries affected, and that *sanitary cordon* was a meaningless expression because it was neither practicable nor possible to establish a rigid line along thousands of kilometres of the frontier. In all the recommendations and reports presented and approved by the Conference, therefore, the expression *sanitary zone* substituted for *sanitary cordon* and *stations of exchange or observation* for *quarantine stations*.

Along the final part of his report Rajchman explained the definite plan of campaign. He reminded the Conference that it had recognized that the defensive policy of strengthening the system of sanitary organization established on the Western frontiers of Russia by her neighbours was not sufficient. The alternative plan of simply extending this organization to the Russian side of the border, and of thus establishing a double system of sanitary barriers on both sides of the frontiers, had also been considered inadequate, and the Conference had proposed that, in addition to these defensive measures, a concerted attack should be carried out on the epidemics at their source. It had, however, been thought impracticable to draw up a plan of action covering the whole of Russia and the Ukraine. It would require huge, unattainable funds, and could not be carried out with the sanitary staff available in the countries involved.[19]

The Conference had decided, therefore, that the offensive part of the program should be confined to railways and waterways and to a selected area within Russia, which was of vital importance for the economy and trade of Russia and the Ukraine. In the annexes to the report of the Third Committee it had been proposed tentatively that the Donctz Basin should be dealt with in this way, for the following specific reasons:

1. The coal and iron-ore mines of Russia were concentrated there.
2. It was an epidemic centre of typhus and cholera.
3. It was a famine area and had an easy access through several Black Sea ports.

The Conference had not only recommended a technical program of action along the region, but had also suggested to the governments principles on which this action should be based. Eight proposals had been adopted which emphasized the necessity for the participation of all the European Governments. In addition, a definite scale for apportioning the expenses had been laid down. The Conference had decided what control should be provided, and had suggested the organization to which the execution of its recommendations should be entrusted, while insisting on the necessity of the action itself being left in the hands of the Public Health Services of the countries concerned.

It had been at this stage that the only differences of opinion in the Conference had openly arisen. Rajchman emphasized the fact that the technical report, i.e. the constructive and technical part of the proposals, had been accepted unanimously by all the Delegations without any exception whatever. Although the question of what international body should be entrusted with the supervision of the work raised a difference of opinion, the spirit of conciliation and mutual understanding so prominent a feature of the Conference, the two Delegations who found themselves in the minority framed a resolution in an extremely conciliatory spirit. Therefore, the Conference as a whole had immediately agreed to present the views of these two Delegations as a minority resolution, together with the proposals of the twenty-five remaining national Delegations.

The final conclusions of the Conference would be presented, together with the report of the proceedings, to the Genova Conference, through the intermediary of the Council of the League of Nations. Rajchman had no doubt that the Delegates would use their influence within their governments in order to persuade them to adopt these recommendations when these governments met, no later than in two or three weeks' time, to give the final sanction to the work of the Warsaw Conference.

The International Health Board of the Rockefeller Foundation gets Involved

On 18 February 1922 Ludwik Rajchman sent an extensive report to the Delegate of the European Office of the Rockefeller Foundation in Paris, Wickliffe Rose. Within this report he discussed the hard epidemic situation in Eastern Europe.[20] It had been issued to all State Members and the Polish Government had applied officially for immediate convocation of the expert European Conference in Warsaw to consider the situation, concerting measures to be taken to prevent infection from spreading westwards and a plan for stabilizing a *sanitary belt* (or sanitary zones) on both sides of the frontier between Russia and the Ukraine on the one side, and Poland and Rumania on the other. Technical representatives of twenty European Governments attended the Warsaw conference; the US Public Health also being represented. It took four months before succeeding in bringing together the Polish and Russian delegates to the conference table, but, instead of diplomatic difficulties, closer cooperation resulted between the Russian and Polish health authorities. According to Rajchman, 'the question now will be to obtain general agreement for the establishment of this sanitary belt. In our mind it should consist of concentric lines, epidemic hospitals, quarantine and feeding stations, public bath, and delousing establishments, etc. on both sides of the frontier to a depth of some 150 km'.[21] Special courses were organized for training the staff engaged in the campaign, and sanitary agreements were concluded between the countries of Eastern Europe. The main target was preserving Central Europe from the hazard represented by the spread of the epidemics.[22]

This strategy, supported by the members of the expert commission on Epidemics, was to be maintained by governments, but they were unable to do it with their own resources. Rajchman insisted in front of the Rockefeller authorities on the fact that the anti-typhus campaign in Poland was considered to be the first successful effort in Europe in international public health work. However he was afraid about epidemics getting out of control and he proposed taking W. Rose to the conference as a unique opportunity to get in contact with representatives of European delegations to build a permanent organizing effort involving the expertise and resources of the Rockefeller Foundation.[23] Since this dramatic situation in the early 1920s and onwards, aggravated by malnutrition and a critical recoil in the living standards, the technical advice and the collaboration of the RF was permanent in epidemic campaigns and especially in the fight against malaria, trachoma and other social diseases affecting specific regions of Europe.[24]

In the latter part of 1921, famine appeared on an enormous scale in Russia and emigration of populations from the stricken regions added hundreds of thousands of Polish war refugees seeking repatriation. The extreme situation was the cause of the violent recrudescence of typhus, accompanied by relapsing fever and cholera. The situation was out of control when the Health Section undertook to supply this need, international experts were sent to the field and international working groups were established with government health authorities and voluntary agencies acting into the field. Epidemiological information was received from areas involved and government health services were supported to challenge what proved to be an epidemic of typhus, relapsing fever and cholera of overwhelming proportion, sweeping westward from the famine-stricken regions of Russia and the Ukraine.[25]

The Warsaw conference formulated plans for sanitary interventions to provide mutual exchange of information and the coordination between neighbouring countries to prevent the spread of the infections, drafting a campaign and appealing the governments of all European countries to provide funds at about $600,000, entrusting the Health Organization with the execution of the plan.[26]

On 18 April 1922 Rajchman issued to Rose his report on the *Warsaw European Health Conference,* held under the auspices of the League of Nations. He considered the epidemic situation as a matter of international sanitary concern, and therefore he tried to involve the authorities of the Rockefeller Foundation. The funds available for the interventions proposed were not enough to fulfil the program to be carried out. Conventions on quarantines and sanitary arrangements were approved and the application of resolutions was left to the Epidemic Commission of the League of Nations. In addition, one of the most relevant collaborative programmes, the creation of an *International Epidemiological Intelligence Service* funded by the Rockefeller Foundation, was proposed in the frame of this Conference felt as a necessity for the evaluation of any case prior to an international intervention.

In this inter-governmental collaboration to overcome the epidemic threat the main coordinating efforts were conducted by the Epidemic Commission of the League trying to assist Public Health Services in Eastern Europe in the fight against the epidemic of typhus. A Commission consisting of Thorvald Madsen, Director of the Staten Serum Institute, Copenhagen, appointed President of the Health Committee of the League of Nations; George Buchanan, Senior Medical Officer at the British Ministry of Health, appointed as Vice-President of the

Health Committee of the League of Nations; J. Jitta, President of the Hygiene Council at the Low Countries; Ricardo Jorge, Director General, Portuguese Public Health Administration; and Dr Violle, Pasteur Institute, worked together publishing a report for the preparation of a new International Sanitary Convention for the study of existing quarantine arrangements and new agreements.

Under those exceptional circumstances, the sanitary situation in Eastern Europe had attracted interest of the Rockefeller Foundation. In 1922 Rose published an assessment of the epidemic situation summarizing the role of the Rockefeller Foundation and the League of Nations.[27] As soon as early 1919 attention was called to an appalling epidemic of typhus, which was sweeping over Russia and Poland as a result of war and post-war conditions involving extensive territories inhabited by millions of people. The government administrative machinery, including sanitary organization and campaigns, had broken down and the two countries were still at war. The movement of armies and refugees along huge territories spread the epidemics and added difficulties to the implementation of any measures of control. The situation represented a serious hazard to the population concerned, as well as to the surrounding countries. Relief agencies supported by volunteers proved unable to handle the problem and when it became evident that the fight against the epidemic involved provisions of food, clothing and shelter on a scale which only governments and international aid could undertake; an official appeal was made to the League of Nations for intervention.

This was the origin of the international intervention. Early in 1920, the Council of the League requested to all interested governments for funds and appointed an international Epidemic Commission to manage such funds as might be convenient.[28] During the first year the commission worked in closed association with the governments directly concerned and demonstrated its usefulness as an agency for effective international cooperation. Cases of typhus fell in Poland from 157,000 in 1919 to 45,000 in 1921, and in Russia from about 3,000,000 to 600,000 and in Romania from 45,555 to 4,834.

During the autumn of 1922 the technical support of the Epidemic Commission was also required to challenge the huge problem of refugees in Greece. More than 750,000 refugees from Asia Minor were moved as a consequence of the advance of the Turkish troops. Cases of smallpox, cholera and typhoid fever had been declared and a wide vaccination campaign was organized by the Epidemic Commission with the aid of Greek doctors and public health inspectors to attend 550,000 refugees. Emergence intervention to cope with pandemics became essential by the 1920s.

During the following months the epidemic situation in Eastern Europe became greatly impaired as a result of the famine in Russia, and the health status of the population increasingly became an international political problem. It is worthwhile to retain that while the League of Nations Epidemic Commission was carrying out these urgent tasks in 1922, a provisional Health Committee was being approved at

Geneva. Epidemics and malnutrition in Eastern Europe were not considered yet as a huge political problem, notwithstanding the big efforts implemented in the fight by the Health Organization, and was still considered on a provisional basis. The third Assembly of the League of Nations had to decide in September 1922 whether a permanent status should be given to it and the program of work. Obviously, the permanent collaborative agreements with the RF were in favour of its persistence.

The public health expert Hans Zinsser did a journey as a member of the Epidemic Commission of the Health Section of the League of Nations to Russia between the 11 June and 20 July 1923, issuing a detailed report to the League health authorities.[29] He followed instructions from Rajchman to survey the experiment of vaccination by the method recommended by the French bacteriologist Alexander Mikhailovich Besredka, born in Odessa, a pupil of Ilya Metchnikov at the Pasteur Institute who had become a French citizen in 1910. Immediately the possibility of participation by the League in the future control of the cholera epidemics in Russia was requested. Zinsser spent three weeks in Russia, most of the time around Moscow and making a trip to Postov and to Khartov.

The work began by a discussion meeting with Dr Panataleoni, President of the Epidemic Commission, about the main problems to challenge. Zinsser met a series of Russian experts: Siemashko, Syassin and Professors Barykin, Korshun and Lubarski of the Russian Scientific Commission on Vaccination. His report was divided into two topics: the experiments on vaccination that were taking place and the epidemiological control of cholera, considering both the localization of cases and the possibility of establishing a European barrier to prevent the disease.[30]

Before Zinsser's visit in 1923, a considerable amount of work had been carried out in Russia on vaccination per os (oral administration). The Russian Government had appointed a scientific commission and the vaccination was almost completed in 1923. The vaccines used were largely manufactured by Russian laboratories, some of them in the form of tablets and others like a liquid vaccine consisting of cholera cultures precipitated with 20 per cent alcohol. A preliminary conference of experts took place upon the arrival of Zinsser and after the meeting he deduced that the difficulties of carrying out the vaccination experiment under the prevailing conditions: the variety of vaccines employed, the lack of bile and limited facilities rendered unlikely a uniform perspective of the vaccination campaign, lacking of an efficient coordination.[31]

After a discussion of a detailed vaccination plan, on 13 July a plenary session took place and the plan of procedure for vaccination was unanimously adopted. It was accepted that a separate group of experiments should be made for each of the diseases to be studied, namely cholera, typhoid fever and dysentery. It was decided that in certain chosen localities it would be of advantage to carry out the experiments in a considerable number of different sections of the Russian Federation, since sanitary and climatic conditions were substantially different and this factor influenced the course of epidemics. However, wherever vaccination was carried out no less than 1,000 people in each place were to be vaccinated in order to concentrate the records. It was agreed that whenever possible the experiments should be carried out in places affected by epidemics or those in absence of epidemics in which the study of the preceding year indicated the likelihood of an increasing sick-rate for the summer months. The experts selected age groups between 18 and 45 years, excluding the very young and the aged sectors of the population, starting the vaccination campaigns within one month. Each vaccination group was to be placed under the permanent supervision of a local physician and a medical officer had to take care of the general observation of the group. The Russian Vaccination Commission considered that the minimum number was:

> Cholera: 30,000 vaccinations, necessitating 90,000 tablets
> Typhoid: 10,000 vaccinations, necessitating 30,000 tablets
> Dysentery Shiga: 5,000 vaccinations, necessitating 15,000 tablets
> Dysentery Flexner: 5,000 vaccinations, necessitating 15,000 tablets[32]

After a technical discussion about the several varieties of vaccines produced in Russian laboratories the Commission determined that only vaccines prepared under the direction of Professor Besredka or similarly prepared in dry form were to be used. Zinsser was told to submit to Rajchman the request for sufficient number of Besredka tablets of French manufacture and sufficient bile to be used with these tablets.[33] In addition the League of Nations was also requested to pay salaries for doctors involved in the campaigns.

When the purpose of Zinsser's visit to Russia was discussed with Rajchman and the head of the IHB of the Rockefeller Foundation, F. F. Russell in New York, it was considered advisable that a certain amount of attention was given to a more intensive study of the epidemiology of cholera in Russia. The South Eastern provinces were the regions in which endemic foci constituted a permanent threat for all Western European countries. Cholera epidemics in Russia had usually spread from these provinces provoking outbreaks in the Volga area, south from Samara, Saratoff, Tzaritzin and Astrakhan, Rostov and the Caucasia Region.

> It is likely that the distribution of cholera in Russia during the last two years, because of the unusual movement of the population under the pressure of famine, the conditions of troop transportation etc. has been considerably shifted. Indeed, outbreaks were observed a year ago as far north as Archangel, where they were traced to the transportation of 'carriers' from the famine region (personal communication from professor Barykin) and consequent upon such shifting of the population peculiar local conditions have probably led to the centralisation of intense cholera incidence in places where ordinarily cholera is merely sporadic. The enormous sick rate at Odessa in 1922 and similar concentrations in recent years at some other places not usually affected depended most probably upon wretched local sanitary conditions in which even the ordinary protective organisation had broken down in consequence of political an economic emergencies.[34]

Considering the situation, Zinsser estimated pertinent an attempt to determine and measure the extension of the endemic foci, so that a sanitary intervention and an attempt towards their isolation was instituted, and the establishment of a cholera barrier between European Russia and the South East regions. But both projects appeared excessively ambitious and the projects had to be regarded as the beginning of an uncertain long period of efforts. The last part of the scientific program involved the analysis of 'carriers' transmitting the infection. The plan of intervention suggested that in each of the places chosen a cross section of 2,000 to 3,000 people, selected from the most exposed groups, be subjected to medical checking to find out the percentage of positive cases.[35] This plan followed a similar pattern as others developed by the IHB of the Rockefeller Foundation in American and European countries. It would be of epidemiological value during the intervals between epidemic outbreaks. But no plan for a generalized cholera campaign could be complete without an attempt to establish a barrier against the spread of the disease from the endemic regions. The League of Nations Health Section had encouraged for the establishment of a barrier on the Polish border, and the experts considered this could be worked out without much difficulty, although, connected with the scheme schools for sanitary inspectors were necessary.[36] With the initiatives of the Epidemic Commission and the consolidation of the Health Organization of the League, international diplomacy around public health became closely related to the League and the Rockefeller decisions since the early 1920s.

3 THE EXTENSION OF THE COLLABORATIVE PROGRAMME

Interchange of Public Health Experts and Schools of Public Health

The Health Committee of the League of Nations assumed to intervene directly in the instruction of public health experts considering it as a cornerstone to implement health policies both nationally and internationally. This educational work, promoted by the Health Organization of the League, was directly related to previous strategies implemented by the IHB of the RF. A principal aspect for the authorities of the Health Organization was to recognize the importance for public health experts to have information and a wide perspective of how fundamental health problems were dealt with in different countries. The central concept was 'hygiene is primarily a matter of education'[1] and this sentence applied not only to the citizens but also to national authorities and health officers. In order to improve the international coordination, several lines of action were developed in this direction, the first one covering the publication of how health care services were organized and how they operated in different European countries. This included information about sanitary regulations, the technical strategies applied for the identification and measure of social health problems and the public and private institutions involved. In total accordance with the public health ideology and previous strategies developed by the Rockefeller Foundation, the LNHO promoted interchanges between countries by funding visits of public health experts to study and discuss the functioning of health care systems in other countries:

> The organisation of travelling exchanges involving health experts in different countries was an initiative easily developed by the Secretariat of the League of Nations and the health authorities in different countries. The International Health Board of the Rockefeller Foundation assumed the program and contributed with generous grants to those exchange visits, the first of them taking place in October 1922. The plan was settled according to different schemes: some visits were devoted to exchange of public health officers; others, applied to specialists in tuberculosis, children's health, school hygiene, health administrators of harbours, statistical demographers, etc. In 1930, six hundred officers, not only of state members of the League of Nations, but

> also from other non member countries, such as the United States of America, Mexico and the Soviet Union, took part in the exchange visits of sanitary staff. Among the visited nations were most of the European countries, Latin America, United States of America, Canada, Western Africa, India and Japan.[2]

To start with, on 18 November 1921 Ludwik Rajchman, Medical Director of the LNHO, sent a report to the RF entitled *The League of Nations Health Organisation. What it is and How it Works.*[3] As we know, he had previously initiated the negotiations with Wickliffe Rose for a general agreement of collaboration between the League of Nations and the Rockefeller Foundation in specific domains of international health. The agreement was passed by the Council of the League in September 1922, and one of the main issues was the maintenance of an International Interchange of Public Health Personnel on an international scale.

> The Health Organisation of the League of Nations will establish and maintain an International Interchange of Public Health Personnel as a separate branch of its work, to begin operations on October 1st 1922, or as soon thereafter as possible, and to continue for not less than three years unless by mutual agreement between the League of Nations and the Rockefeller Foundation some other arrangement is made.[4]

The work of the Interchange of Public Health Personnel was to be conducted along a series of general lines to bring public health administrators in different countries into closer relationship with each other, making comparative learning, evaluation and management of the organization and legislation on public health. This strategy would contribute to an international perspective of health problems whilst also encouraging the spirit of collaboration. The interchange program endeavoured to obtain the cooperation of the public health administrations for the purpose of agreeing upon a uniform international standard of public health expertise, health politics and regulations. The program was based on the organization of meetings involving the participation of public health officials from various countries, making it possible for these officials to remain for a certain time attached to the health services of their countries, so that they might have opportunities of exchanging views on health problems, acquainting themselves with the public health organizations of those countries with the manner in which the regulations were applied and with the duties of the health officials.

Annual reports of the administration of the Interchange of Public Health Personnel Program were rendered to the Council and to the Assembly of the League of Nations, and copies of these reports were forwarded regularly to the International Health Board/Division of the Rockefeller Foundation. Moreover, representatives of the Rockefeller Foundation were kept closely and regularly informed of the activities of the personnel interchange and had the opportunity to express their points of view and their criticism.

Convinced of the effectiveness of this program, the Rockefeller Foundation agreed to pay an annual subvention to meet the expenses of the Interchange of Public Health Personnel, not to exceed $60,080 a year for each of the three years from 1922 to 1925. Further agreements were made thereafter and, as a matter of fact, the RF continued to support the Interchange program by specific grants until the end of 1931:

October to December 1925	25,000 SF
1926	75,000 SF
1927 to 1931	50,000 SF per year

Table 3.1: **Grant for the Maintenance of the Program of Interchange of Public Health Personnel on an International Scale. Source: Rockefeller Archive Centre.**

The grants for 1930 and 1931 were parts of a consolidate grant expiring on 31 December 1934.[5]

The Rockefeller Foundation agreed to pay the annual subvention in quarterly instalments, beginning 1 October 1922, directly to the Financial Director of the Secretariat of the League of Nations, who was to administer the subvention paid by the Rockefeller Foundation as a separate Fund, to be known as the Interchange of Public Health Personnel Fund. This Fund made disbursements from at the direction of the Secretary-General of the League of Nations, after the budget had to be approved by the Health Organization of the League. The special accounts of the Financial Director for the Interchange of Public Health Personnel Fund was audited as directed by the Council of the League of Nations. Even considering the bureaucratic complexity of the decision making and procedures of approval derived from the plurality of organs involved, in this case, as in the rest of grants contributed by the RF, a thorough and strict monitoring of the use of the money and the budget expenditure took place.

The annual statement of account of the Interchange of Public Health personnel Fund was rendered to the Council and to the Assembly of the League of Nations, and copies of these statements were forwarded regularly to the International Health Board of the Rockefeller Foundation. The Interchange Program was subjected to an Agreement, which might be modified by the mutual consent of the Council of the League of Nations and the Rockefeller authorities. As a matter of fact, the agreement was initially approved by the Council of the League and became effective on their approval by the IHB of the RF.

Wickliffe Rose appreciated this interchange policy of public health experts. The RF considered that a fundamental condition of effective teamwork was mutual acquaintance, understanding and good will, a strategy shown at the international health conferences held by the Health Organization in London and Warsaw to face the huge problems of epidemics in Russia and Poland.[6] Diplomacy was a cornerstone and the role of the League irreplaceable. The Health Committee soon appreciated the opportunity to improve the information, influence the professional training and increase the international experience of public health authorities and health officers in as many countries as possible. The interchange was not conceived for simple observation, but for periods of definite service, establishing helpful contacts as a real exchange of experience on practical issues.

One of the first decisions was the publication and circulation of reports about the organization of public health services and their activities in several European countries. Those reports contained information on the administrative regulations, health legislation, social dominant diseases, implementation of sanitary campaigns and definition of main health problems, as well as the cooperation between private associations and health authorities. The *International Health Yearbook,* issued for the first time in 1925, updated information each year about the progress made in each participating country, new preventive measures implemented, health care facilities and any other measures introduced. We shall discuss the search for an epidemiological internationalization in a further chapter.

Nevertheless, Rajchman was convinced that progress in international hygiene could not be based exclusively on the exchange of information and laboratory research. For the best operation of the scheme on *Interchange of Public Health Officials* the leading authorities of the League proposed to implement the so called *study tours*, holding four times a year a monthly workshop at which fifty Medical Officers of Health, commissioned by ten to fifteen Governments, would meet and be addressed by leading sanitarians. The aim of those study tours undertaken by health officials was to bring hygienists in touch with experts in other countries not only for his personal benefit, but also to promote international cooperation. It is important to keep in mind that health was more and more a matter of political concern and a very attractive issue for insurance companies, the international market and new industrial initiatives. The Medical Officers would then proceed to work within the ranks of another Public Health Administration for a further period of eight weeks. Between 1922 and 1929, $500,000 was provided to put into practice the program of exchange of public health experts.[7] The activities started after a resolution adopted by the Provisional Health Committee of the League at its Third Session held in Paris in May 1922. The resolution was approved in the following terms:

> The Health Committee has taken note of the proposal regarding an interchange of sanitary personnel between different countries interested in its being carried into effect, and, in consideration of the great utility of ensuring that sanitary officers should become acquainted with practical solutions of public health problems as well as the organisation of public health services in various countries, recommends that the necessary steps should be taken by approaching the Governments interested in the matter in order to carry into effect this interchange at least as a provisional and experimental measure.[8]

The first experimental interchange of experts began in October 1922 thanks to the grant delivered by the IHB of the Rockefeller Foundation for this purpose, and the close relation between the League Secretariat and the health authorities in the various countries involved in the experience. The program lasted from October until December 1922, took place in Belgium and Italy and apparently it fulfilled the expectancies of the various health administrations participating.

Since 1923 interchanges were arranged regularly to promote collaboration between health authorities of various countries and to provide opportunities to take advantage of experiences in the organization and administration of public health policies. Implemented in some cases at national level, no international experiences in this sense existed previously, although most of the huge public health problems were not national but international in scope and extent, since hazards do not respect political borders. This was the main argument raised by the defenders of the initiative. Programs for post-graduate instruction was long felt by national and international authorities and keeping an effective public health administration represented a process of continuous adjustment to advances of science, medical technologies and methods of measuring the dimension of the problems. A repeated argument was that although the collective interchange was primarily beneficial for individuals, benefits were supposed in turn to public health services.[9] The program was granted by the IHB of the Rockefeller Foundation and was conceived in several ways: some activities applied for public health officers, others were conceived for specific issues such as policies and campaigns to fight tuberculosis, to promote infant hygiene, to introduce school hygiene, to organize local and national health administration units, such as port stations, and to organize demographic and epidemiologic statistics services.

Selskar Gunn, Director of the IHB RF at the Paris Office by that time, sent periodical reports about the program to the central office of the RF in New York. On 12 October 1923 he wrote F. F. Russell:

> Dr Rajchman was in Paris the last two days. I had several conversations with him. He states that, in general, the first year's experience with the Interchange Health Officials has been very successful and that this kind of activity is now accepted by both the Health Committee of the League of Nations and the Assembly as a valuable part of the work of the League ... The Interchange program for 1924 is to consist of four Collective Interchanges and two Specialists Interchanges. The Collective Interchange will be as follows: 1. England; 2. Holland and Denmark; 3. Switzerland; 4. Far East. Specialist Interchanges will be for tuberculosis officers and school medical inspectors. It is anticipated for each of the Collective Interchanges that approximately twenty men will participate, and for each of the Specialist Interchanges ten men.[10]

The first interchanges were assessed as successful. However, on 14 February 1924, Gunn reported to Russell some difficulties affecting the Interchange Program: 'Rajchman finds now himself in an extremely difficult situation because of the enormous increase in the cost of travelling ... Dr Rajchman believes that it will be necessary for him to abandon the interchange of port officers in the Far East and probably also de interchange of medical school officers'.[11]

The specific initiatives planned by Rajchman for 1924 were:

1. Malaria interchanges involving six to eight expert malariologists.
2. Interchange of Medical Officers of large urban areas. The proposal came from England and the suggestion was that the Chief Medical Officer were involved and accompanied by the Head of the Department of Housing.
3. Enlargement of the plan of individual missions.
4. A series of collective studies applied for small groups of specialists sent for particular investigations: i.e. for the evaluation of communicable diseases, particularly scarlet fever and diphtheria.

It was imperative assessing the situation in each case and situation. Health policies were very different and, for instance, some countries were spending huge sums of money for the isolation of hospitals while others spent very little. All the four initiatives for the program were to receive an amount of $10,500 each, reaching the total budget $42,000.

On March 13, 1924 Russell sent a critical answer to Gunn, requesting a closer control of the development of the program:

> I am as you know entirely sympathetic with the work in which Doctor Rajchman and the Health Committee are engaged ... [but] You must investigate further in order to see if a conference of leading malariologists would be justified; who might attend, where and when, and under which auspices it could be held and what the expenses would be ... In the present letter you estimate that 10,500 $ would be needed. That seems rather large for one, fairly short meeting to be attended by a few men.[12]

Indeed Russell showed some doubts about the future of the Program of Interchanges of Health Personnel and proposed to consider the initiative as a part of the fellowship program.[13] Nevertheless the interchange followed year after year and was presented as one of the most successful initiatives of the HO. Creating a well structured network of leaders in public health was hard and expensive, but it gave visibility and capacity of influence to the League and the RF International Health Board. Gunn sent periodical detailed information to Russell after the reports transmitted by Rajchman about the evolution of the several parts of the program.

As a matter of fact, the Conference of Malariologists (1924) gathered the most relevant international experts on malaria policies and research. A. Lutrario acted as chairman, and B. Nocht, L. Raynaud, D. Ottolenghi, G. Pittaluga and Colonel James were some of the prominent participants. Other corresponding members from affected countries were also present: N. H. Swellengrebel and Marcinowski (Russia), Sfarcic (Yugoslavia) among other malariologists from

Poland, Bulgaria, Rumania and Greece. N. Lothian and G. Druetti, members of the Health Section, acted as technical secretaries. Independently of the collaboration agreement, the RF showed a permanent interest about the activities promoted by the Health Organization regarding malaria: meetings, technical reports, interchange experiences, preventing campaigns and therapeutic initiatives. The RF leaders received very detailed information about the activities boosted by the experts of the HO on the field of malaria.

Gunn was the transmitter to the New York Rockefeller leaders of the arguments stated by Rajchman for the continuation of the programs. He assumed that his arguments were worthy, being a fact that the financial situation in Europe was still very difficult after the war years. He showed himself in favour of a larger appropriation for Interchange during the following two years, being convinced of the value of this activity, taking into account that the League still considered Interchange as a permanent part of the program of the Health Section.

In September 1924 Rajchman informed Gunn that 'The Health Committee is now definitively convinced that the system of exchanges has given proof of its practical value ... The object of these interchanges is to enable the participants to acquire technical knowledge by getting into touch with Public Health Administrations in the countries of which they are the guests, and, by this means to create a spirit of mutual understanding and cooperation'.[14] Therefore the Committee for Financial Questions decided that the budget allocation for interchange should be increased during 1925 from 50,000 to 150,000 SF.

The Interchange Program of Health Officials arranged by the Health Section from March to May 1925 was very ambitious. It involved major cities of the United States of America such as Baltimore, New York City and others in Louisiana, Mississippi, Alabama and Washington. The working points included rural health and municipal sanitation, malaria research and anti-malaria campaigns, industrial plants, education in public health, welfare institutions, health administration, the fight against typhoid fever and hookworm control, visits to the Johns Hopkins programs in public health and sanitation, children's health including children's bureau and children hospitals, veterinary inspection, management of slaughter houses, quarantine stations, immigration examinations and health facilities. The list of guests participating in the scientific tour was composed of representatives of American countries: Louis Destouches (League of Nations), Alberto Zwanck (Argentina), Emygdio José de Mattos (Brazil), Rafael Álvarez (Cuba), Pedro de Alba Álvarez (México), Andrés Gubetich (Paraguay), Juan Francisco Valega (Perú), Carlos Lardé-Arthès (Salvador), Rafael Schiaffino (Uruguay), Leopoldo García Maldonado (Venezuela), together with thirty-eight guests belonging to the USA institutions participating. The tour was clearly focused on involving Latin American leaders on public health intervention.

Generally speaking, after a period of five years the program had been improved, the best candidates were selected for each case and a careful preparation of each interchange was planned. The national characteristics of the public health systems were explained and the visiting group was divided into sections consisting of two or three public health officers devoted to routine study of a particular health department without disturbing its normal functioning. Pamphlets describing the activities and departments were distributed in advance to the participants with valuable information concerning the organization of the various public health services.

Various types of collective interchanges were organized, the most common being that of health officers. Others which were more specific, focused on particular issues, gathered specialists such as health officers of maritime stations on the Mediterranean and Baltic areas, tuberculosis officers, sanitary engineers, medical school inspectors and some others. In addition, two international courses in public health were also organized, the first one in Paris for public health officers familiar with French language and the second one in London (November 1927). These courses aimed at the instruction of public health officers by leading specialists of public health administrations. After the lectures, participants studied practical methods of implementation in selected districts of particular countries.

The malaria courses were an offshoot of this system of interchanges. Trained experts were needed in a number of countries and the League boosted malaria courses at national health institutes in Hamburg, London and Paris complemented with practical training activities in the field in Italy, Spain and Yugoslavia.

As a general working philosophy, the countries where the interchange was held always assumed a part of the expense. Travel expenses and hotel expenses were normally assumed by the governments involved in the interchanges, and the cost of instruction was partially funded by the League. Sometimes Governments contributed to manage the expense by sending participants at the cost of their own administration. This practice became more common and, for the malaria courses held in 1926, more than half of the forty-seven participants attended at the expense of their own administration. The expenses assumed by the Health Organization were debited to the credits placed by the League and the grants of the IHD of the Rockefeller Foundation. The League started the program placing 50,000 SF in 1923, increasing to 150,000 SF during the following years. In addition about one third of the total expenses were paid by governments and participants.[15]

Despite the achievements the program was not exempt of diplomatic tensions, as it may have been expected under such complex international situation. The Government of Colombia complained about its exclusion regretting that a delegate from Colombia had not been invited to participate in the Interchange of Health Officials to visit the public health facilities in the USA.[16] 'If we knew here that the Colombian Government had been officially invited to submit the name of a candidate for this last interchange I am sure that it might ease the feelings of certain health officials and others interested in public health who are now wondering why Colombia was not included'.[17]

The program for 1926 included collective interchanges in Great Britain and Denmark.[18] The interchanges in Great Britain were restricted to municipal health officers and visits were made to London institutions and the counties. An Interchange of Sanitary Engineers was planned in London at the same time involving the assistance of members of the Royal Sanitary Institute for that purpose. The Collective Interchange in Denmark was shaped as the usual type and candidates were secured as a rule from agricultural countries. The Interchange on the West Coast of Africa began in March and included participants from the Colonies in that area and three from Latin America, a region whose health officers took part as well in the Collective Interchanges in Denmark and Great Britain.

Rajchman prepared next an interchange of a special type in the hope that it would combine the advantages of the individual mission and that of the collective visit, doing away with some of the disadvantages affecting both. The new model of interchange was to be held in July 1926 being restricted to about 10 participants from three or four neighbouring countries. The participants would be general health officers with special interests and special subjects in which two or three of the participant countries were affected. Therefore the issues would be locally analyzed, although the whole group would work together for the consideration of problems interesting all them. In addition, an Interchange of officers from maritime health stations in the Baltic area was under consideration. The initiative was similar to the Interchange of Maritime Health Officers in the Mediterranean area which began on 10 November 1926.[19]

The program was successful although some controversial attitudes appeared from time to time. Gunn maintained an interview with the public health expert and Yugoslavian authority Andreja Stampar – director of the Zagreb School of Public Health and member of the League, professor of hygiene at the Zagreb University and fellow of the RF – about the Interchange of physicians from the League of Nations in Yugoslavia since 18 May to 1 July.[20] Unfortunately Gunn reported Stampar's criticism and discomfort regarding some aspects of the organization and attitudes of the participants:

> He wonders on what basis the Interchange men are chosen. From the 16 men now in Yugoslavia he states that two possess some intelligence; he did not mention which two. Most of them are not only stupid, but even if they learnt something in Yugoslavia, they are so far down the scale in rank and office that they could not put their knowledge into action. He says that there are no directors of public health or directors of laboratories among the group; that is men who have some power and influence in their own countries, and he does not understand just where he is going to accomplish anything showing County health officers from other countries the Yugoslav organization when these men have no chance of profiting because of the small positions which they hold. There have also been some disagreeable incidents, which have

> made Dr. Stampar rather antagonistic to the Interchange. One man, I did not say who, rides around from place to place in the automobile of the Ministry of Health ... Another, a German representative, drinks no less than three litres of wine daily. A third, a French representative brought his wife and little child along and is making a holiday of the trip, insisting that the League of Nations must pay the travelling expenses of his family. Dr Stampar said he would not do this, and the hotel bill which is still due will probably be paid by the Yugoslav Ministry in the end.[21]

Gunn considered in his internal report that perhaps Stampar was a bit unreasonable due to a few personal things, which had arisen. Nevertheless he was so emphatic that there must be something in his complaining.[22] According to Rajchman, Stampar had exaggerated a good deal. After a further conversation between Stampar and Gunn, he changed his mind showing a more flexible attitude. Nevertheless, this incident was exceptional among the general feeling of satisfaction.

During the period 1922 to 1927 collective interchanges were held in a wide series of territories worldwide: Algeria, Austria, Belgium, Canada, Cuba, Czechoslovakia, Dahomey, Danzig, Denmark, Egypt, France, Gambia, Germany, Gold Coast, Great Britain, Greece, French Guinea, Portuguese Guinea, Hungary, Italy, Ivory Coast, Japan, Korea, Latvia, Manchuria, the Netherlands, Nigeria, Norway, Palestine, Poland, Senegal, Kingdom of the Serbs, Croats and Slovenes, Sierra Leone, Spain, Sudan, Sweden, Switzerland, Syria, Togoland and the United States of America.[23] The participants in the activities were drawn from fifty-two countries, thirteen colonies or protectorates and two mandates territories. In addition fifty-seven medical officers from thirty countries were selected to study certain pressing problems on an individual bases. Experts from Asia were enabled to study the method of preparing and administering anti-cholera vaccines in the countries and laboratories where these methods were developed. In addition, Japanese experts in nutrition were given the opportunity to study advances in the science of nutrition as it was developed in Western laboratories, and specialists in certain branches of public health administration examined certain new methods in other countries.

According to the reports prepared by the League, by 1930, 'six hundred officials belonging to State Members of the League, and also to certain non-member States – such as the United States of America, Mexico, and the USSR – had participated in these interchanges of health personnel. Nearly all countries in Europe, as well as Latin America, the United States, Canada, West Africa, India and Japan, have been visited and have sent their officials to the study tours'.[24] The capacity of influence and networking of the program showed to be huge and very influential.

In the majority of countries, public health work was developed according to national programs and national traditions. Therefore, the exchange of experience on an international scale was not usual and had the good consequence of opening new initiatives. Nevertheless, the Health Organization of the League, assessing the practical consequences of the program, complained about the fact that the information and experience acquired in one country was not available to others in such a practical way as to avoid the expense of repeating the mistakes of the pioneers.[25] This resistance showed to have even more inefficient consequences considering the main justification of the initiative: public health problems do not have a national scope and extent, demanding campaigns against hazards, which should not be limited to political boundaries. The ideology inherent to the program was evident: well-trained public health officers were in a position to derive great profit from opportunities of collective study of the methods and practices in other countries. It seemed evident that when new public health services were put to work and required recruiting experts, many of the officers lacked the necessary training and, in such cases, visits and experience at health agencies were of great value. The end of the war had led to the setting of new governments, which were obliged to assume public health services on a large scale, dealing with important social and health problems with relatively untrained staff and evident lack of facilities.[26]

As it has been mentioned above, in addition to the collective interchanges, a great deal of individual missions were organized as well to take health officers to other countries, where local authorities arranged a program of instruction with the participation of local experts. In such individual cases the program consisted of a period of instruction taking into account the health conditions prevailing in the officer's country and its pressing demands. Those interchanges strengthened ties and collaboration between European countries and distant countries from Latin America, India and Japan. The individual mission was designed to meet special conditions. A particular subject might be highly developed in a given country, and it might be desirable for public health officers from another nation to study the new work on the field and take advantage of the developments. Thus the poverty of certain states, and the necessity of reducing the expenses, led to the application of preventive measures by health insurance companies and to the study of the financial dimension of public health to coordinate efforts and prevent wastage. The interchange of experiences on that field was considered to be essential and highly fruitful.

> In the field of health insurance, new systems are being introduced in France, Belgium and Japan, and in Austria and Czechoslovakia important changes are being made in the present systems. In the field of preventive medicine it is important that these countries should study the experience of other countries which have achieved good results, and the individual missions of a well-informed public health official, according to a program prepared by the Health Organisation and the competent authorities of the country to be visited are the best means to this end.[27]

In addition, the exchange of technically competent public health officers could help when dealing with specific problems as it had happened between Brazil and Japan. Public health authorities of Brazil feared immigrants from Japan could spread certain parasitic diseases not well known to Brazilian parasitologists.

Arrangements were made by the Health Organization for a Japanese parasitologist to visit Brazil and study the subject in a Brazilian Institute and for a Brazilian parasitologist to carry on similar studies in Japan. The way was paved for an understanding avoiding restrictive laws and diplomatic conflicts.[28]

In order to promote international cooperation in technical questions related to health problems, two international courses of higher instruction for public health experts were organized in Paris and London in 1927. Medical officers from twenty different nationalities attended the courses taught by lecturers from all over the world and then participated in a practical training tour in a large number of European countries. The system proved very positive especially in particular fields such as the fight against malaria. In such cases regular field courses of training were organized in other countries for the medical officers who were to direct the new or reorganized health services.[29]

The interchange program was maintained during the whole period of collaboration between both institutions, the RF and the LNHO, creating a wide network of exchanges and positive interactions. Between 1923 and 1931 the Health Organization organized thirty-five collective study interchanges, involving thirty-one countries and with the participation of 587 health officers coming from sixty-one countries.[30]

The provisional scheme of interchanges for 1925 included general interchanges to Great Britain, Belgium, Yugoslavia and Japan. Moreover a special plan of interchanges involved specialists visiting Sweden, Russia and France. For 1926 the program consisted on collective interchanges in Great Britain and Denmark. The interchanges in Great Britain were restricted to municipal health officers. An Interchange of Sanitary Engineers was held also in London at the same time with assistance of members of the Royal Sanitary Institute. The Collective Interchange in Denmark conformed to the usual type and candidates were secured as a rule from agricultural countries. The Interchange on the West Coast of Africa began in March 1926, including participants from the Colonies in that area and three Latin American Health Officers, who also took part in the Collective Interchanges in Denmark and Great Britain.[31] Public health and modern experimental medicine circulated fast worldwide boosted by the RF – LNHO interchange program.

An Interchange of a special type started to take place in 1926 being organized in the hope to combine the advantages of the individual missions and of the collective visits as well. This interchange was devoted to general health officers with special interests, being restricted to about ten participants from three or four neighbouring countries. In 1926 two interchanges involving Maritime Health Officers from the Baltic area and Maritime Health Officers in the Mediterranean area took place.[32]

With the expansion of the interchanges and the general involvement of the political administrations, the public health expert became the cornerstone of national and international health policies, a powerful instrument to guarantee the implementation of new organizational schemes, the introduction of new technologies and the legitimation of political action and decisions making. Basically, in this and in other programs the LNHO depended on the RF funds: between a third and a half of the total budget came from the RF. Between 1922 and 1929, the RF provided $500,000 to promote the program of public health experts interchange.[33]

In 1928 a renegotiation of grants and budget took place in order to guarantee the continuation of the program. At the end of this year the IHD of the Rockefeller Foundation had collaborated for more than six years supporting this program and the RF leaders were reluctant to persist in funding it, not because they were critical with the positive results, but because they were contrary to persist financing projects for over five years. However the target of the interchanges system was not reached in 1928 in view of the increasing demands, the good results achieved and the greater efficiency in the organization. After the financial crash in 1929 and during the deep depression that followed, Rajchman made all the possible efforts to convince the RF leaders to maintain the collaboration of the IHD, at least on a scale which allowed the continuity and improvement of this program. Rajchman's arguments were finally convincing.

When the interchange program was again evaluated in 1931 one of the most appreciated achievements was having brought the health services of different countries into closer relationship with each other, facilitating the carrying out of comparative studies about the health organization and legislation in different countries. The organization of every interchange included the preparation of a handbook of the medical and health services of the visited country and the reports, which the participants were requested to prepare, were always comparative studies. Another purpose was obtaining cooperation between public health services to secure agreement upon a uniform standard of public health and health regulations.[34]

Schools of Public Health

Following the strategy of building a strong international network of experts sharing public health knowledge and collaborating in public health policies, as early as January 1923 the Health Committee of the League of Nations agreed to survey the state of the programs of specialization in public health and preventive medicine in European, Japanese and American universities; those experts being the key element of the health administration. On 20 February 1924, the Health Committee created a permanent *Commission on Education in Hygiene and Preventive Medicine*, presided by the French expert Léon Bernard together with seven members. In 1930 the dean of the Medical School in Shanghai joined the commission. Soon after its constitution, the commission decided to make a comparative report on three main topics:

1. Training of experts, considering under that denomination medical officers, engineers, architects, nurses and public health staff.
2. Public health teaching programs devoted to medical students and general practitioners.
3. Public health instruction devoted to social agents such as teachers, priests, civil servants, curators and any other possible agents able to contribute in health education and popularization of hygiene among the population.

The *Commission* designed a project to extend and improve the instruction given at the medical centres, promoting programs for experts in schools of public health, as well as systems of evaluation, preparation of teaching materials for professionals, propaganda measures, popularization programs and the programs to teach hygiene at school. Through the *Commission on Education in Hygiene*, established in 1925, cooperation started with national institutions devoted to instruct public health officers, nurses and auxiliary personnel in most European countries under the responsibility of National Institutes of Hygiene.[35] Since the living conditions and the health indicators in each country were the primary consideration, there was no question of a unique program suitable for all institutes of hygiene, but it seemed a good initiative to give the directors of national institutes of health an opportunity of meeting, discussing problems, exchanging experiences and searching for similar solutions.

A wide series of reports were issued about the situation of public health instruction in Austria, Finland, France, Germany, Hungary, Italy, the United States of America and Yugoslavia.[36] Other reports by Janiszewski showed the situation in Poland, Jitta reported on the Low Countries and Nocht dealt with Germany. The general overview was complemented by other presentations on Belgium (Timbal), France (Léon Bernard), Switzerland and Italy (Ottolenghi), Great Britain (George Newman) and Germany (Carl Prausnitz).[37] The vast amount of information collected by the Committee gave way to a series of publications and international conferences to coordinate strategies in the instruction of experts and strategies of intervention in an international context. Obviously, decisions were not imposed over the states but negotiated under the umbrella of the League of Nations and the growing international influence of the *expert authority*.

In 1926 the first International Conference took place in Warsaw just after the inauguration of the Polish National School of Health. In 1927 a second Conference was held in Budapest and Zagreb on the occasion of the official opening of national schools in Hungary and Yugoslavia. The directors of national schools of Prague, Warsaw, Rio de Janeiro, Sao Paolo and experts of health institutes in London, Berlin, Paris and Bologna took part in the meeting, as well as representatives of the International Health Division of the Rockefeller Foundation and the Johns Hopkins School of Public Health in Baltimore.

The fundamental topic in the agenda was the discussion around the most convenient curriculum for the instruction of public health experts active in national institutions. A discussion and a complex negotiation started around the need of experimental and non-experimental disciplines in the curriculum, the place of statistical knowledge, the importance of the standardization of methods of research in social sciences and the organization of a period of practical training in the field. Public health experts were considered to be the main agents for the planification and implementation of health policies in a context in which preventive action was called to be the cornerstone. Also the state of teaching preventive medicine in the medical curriculum was compared among the different countries and discussed. A general coincidence arose concluding that it was, in general, deeply deficient. The meeting not only focused on education in public health; arrangements were also made for technical cooperation on specific questions such as safe drinking water supplies in rural districts, campaigns of oral vaccination against typhoid fever for children, prevention and treatment of scarlet fever and fight against other infectious diseases.[38]

Training activities reached different levels and included several fields. In some cases, highly specialized courses for experts were organized to update and improve technical skills. This was the case of malaria. The Malaria Commission organized regular courses in malariology in four European universities. All these educational activities were strongly supported considering that the benefits were not for individuals taking part in the programs. Medical students' instruction was also improved, as those issues were included in the programs of the universities in which the experts taught, giving better and more updated information to medical professionals and boosting preventive campaigns by the health administration.

The interchange of public health schools, organized in 1928 for the study of rural hygiene led directly to the convening of a European Conference on Rural Hygiene organized by the League of Nations.[39] The recommendations of that Conference constituted an agreement by the health authorities of European countries on a uniform standard of public health and health regulations in rural districts in the fields of medical care, methods of health organization, drinking water supplies and sewage disposal, housing and land improvement. The conclusions were the core of the debates raised at the European Conference of Rural Health.[40]

This conference was seen with interest by the RF and by the public health authorities at the United States of America because it dealt with subjects, which preoccupied American authorities, sociologists and sanitarians.[41] The first item on the agenda, guiding principles and suitable methods for ensuring effective medical assistance in rural communities, was particularly suitable for USA, as introducing into the state legislatures bills providing for various forms of health insurance was an old claim of a large group of American citizens. Those initiatives were opposed at the time by physicians and medical associations and by other groups including insurance companies. An old conflict of interest that seems to still be alive today. The increasing extent to which local and state health departments were providing for the health care of the patients also met with much opposition from the medical professionals. The insistence of political authorities, sociologists and hygienists that the benefits of modern medicine should be more generally extended to the whole population, to people of all social groups, resulted in the creation of an important national committee in the US presided over by Ray Lyman Wilbur.

The conclusions of the Rural Health Conference as regarding housing was also of considerable interests to the USA:

> The work of the Rockefeller Foundation has resulted in the permeation of European health practice by American influences. The young officials with American training are playing an increasingly important part, and their influence is multiplied by the graduates of the new schools of hygiene. In the smaller countries of Central and Eastern Europe American Public Health practice is almost idealised. On the other hand, in England, Germany, Holland and the Scandinavian countries American influence is much less potent.[42]

American influence in regards to sanitary engineering was particularly strong because in European countries the general practitioner of sanitary engineering was almost non-existent; the engineers working in the health administration were often specialists in rather narrow fields. Consequently, the Rockefeller grants-in-aid to the League's Health Organization permitted the League to employ American public health experts and to undertake work which, in some respects, was distinctly American.[43] According to Boudreau's perception, the conclusions and recommendations of the Conference were greatly influenced by American expertise and practice.[44]

The two most transcendental conferences of directors of national schools of public health took place in Paris and Dresden in 1930. One of the topics discussed was the relation between national schools of health as a place of instruction, and the universities' system and health authorities or public administration. As a starting point, a report contributed by Welch showed the plurality of situations in each country and proposed three principles of action: collaboration between the three institutions – schools of public health, universities and health administration – participation of university representatives and health authorities in the managing boards of the schools and the combination of science and research with a practical engagement to cope with the practical requirements of the population.

The third international meeting of directors of schools of public health took place in Paris in 1930. The conference had a main target: international homologation of the teaching pattern and the professional profile of the national schools of health regarding public health experts.[45] In July 1930 a new conference of European directors of public health schools took place in Dresden, focusing on establishing a minimum common program of training for health officers and the content of teaching preventive and social medicine to medical students. A sub-committee devoted to analyzing the role of public health museums in the vulgarization of hygiene was also established.

The prospective action promoted by the LN and funded by the RF gathered a great deal of information, which helped to discuss the professional profile of the public health expert and the role of health officers in the health administration. Once more the RF contributed technical aid, grants, funds and an integrative international framework. Although the institutional autonomy and the national independence was always recognized and apparently safeguarded, the coordination with health authorities, universities and medical professionals was considered absolutely necessary and increasingly the international context promoted by the HO and the RF put pressure to the national governments. In his final report, Carl Prausnitz insisted on the fundamental difference between experts' knowledge and popularization strategies in language, materials and orientation. The concluding report included five main points under the form of general recommendations:

1 Public Health Schools were essential for the establishment of health policies and for the experts' instruction. Considered as technical institutions, they were to be independent from the administrative structure, political power and university models.
2 During the 1920s a series of institutions shared this profile: the Johns Hopkins School of Public Health in Baltimore, the Harvard School of Public Health in Boston and others, mainly funded by the Rockefeller Foundation. In Europe, national schools were established in Madrid (1924), reformed according with the international standards boosted by the RF IHD in 1930; Warsaw (1925), Budapest and Zagreb (1926), London (1929), Prague (1930) and Athens (1930). The American model was based on specific centres in the frame of prominent universities and the European model usually was based on State institutions. France and Germany followed different patterns, but, in any case, cooperation with the university staff and university teaching and research programs was recognised to be essential.
3 The aim of those institutions, according to Carl Prausnitz's report, was instructing public health experts for the health administration to implement health policies and vulgarising hygiene. They should associate research and teaching, offering practical training as well: laboratory technologies, methods of research in social sciences, popularisation strategies, hygienic education and implementation of sanitary campaigns.
4 Research was an essential task as an expression of the so-called *scientific spirit* attributed to those institutions. But it would not run independent from the practical problems of the population, on the contrary it should go hand in hand to attempt to resolve such problems. In some countries, previous experience showed the positive effects of practical action on specific programs implemented in certain regions.
5 An ambitious proposal was the common agreement about the idea of a common European teaching program to instruct *medical officers of health*.[46]

Moreover, a period of practical training in rural areas for at least three months was recommended as an essential part of the experts' instruction. Students should play an active part in all fields: organizing social hygiene, planning sanitation, taking part in public health administration and drafting programs of hygiene propaganda. States were called to demand the qualification of the National School of Public Health, or a similar institution, from those who applied for an official post in public health services, whether national or municipal. Apparently, this practical training had obtained excellent results in some countries and the leaders of the schools strongly recommended to extend it. As seen, the conferences of directors raised the creation of a professional monopoly associated with public health linked to the public administration.

On the 27 May the League drafted a scheme of the programs for the instruction of public health experts and sent a copy to the IHD of the Rockefeller Foundation.[47] F. F. Russell received the outline of the subjects to be taught in a school of public health as finally adopted by the Paris Conference.[48]

The National Schools of Public Health were designed to monopolize knowledge and expertise, and to legitimate political action and social intervention.[49] Health officers and inspectors were the key element to training medical practitioners, public health assistants and other complementary staff, as well as to advise in popularization campaigns.[50] They were the basic units of public health schools, the site where facilities were to be available to laboratory technologies, instructing lectures, vulgarizing activities and museum materials.

Public Health Schools flourished in the 1920s and 1930s as crucial institutions to coordinate preventive campaigns, organize the fight against social diseases, implement new therapies and vaccination campaigns and legitimating international public health expertise under the impulse of the Rockefeller Foundation IHD and the LNHO. International conferences of directors of public health schools laid down a framework for an international debate about specialization and public health expertise that aimed to shape a pattern of organization, a model of instruction and a coordinated international action, all in accordance to the RF and HO ideas.

Several weeks later, on 27 June 1930, W. H. Howell, director of the Johns Hopkins School of Hygiene and Public Health and one of the participants in the Paris Conference wrote a long letter to the RF leader Russell, containing his personal impressions about the meeting.[51] He realized that there were two different models of organizing the instruction of public health experts. In some countries this depended upon universities and in others it was a responsibility of the central administration. Moreover, the European schools laid more stress upon practical field training, paying less attention to basic instruction and the learning of experimental laboratory methods, as the Americans did. In relation to the situation in Europe, Howell stated:

> they make more of work in what they call social medicine than we do. They define social medicine in vague terms, but it includes health work not only in tuberculosis, venereal diseases, maternal and child welfare, but also in such things as eugenics and alcoholism on which some of them at least laid great stress. As the work on alcoholism was described to me it is much the same as what is attempted in this country by the churches, except that instead of holding over the heads of the delinquents the fear of hell they go strong on the evil results to health, and by persuasion and threats seek to reform their cases.[52]

Howell's words were eloquent. He also expressed his surprise of the rather extraordinary world influence on health work and education that was being exerted by the secretariat of the Health Section of the League of Nations. The directors of all the Continental European Schools of Public Health seemed to rely for guidance upon the officers of the Secretariat, and in the future plans in Greece and in China they had assumed apparently all the responsibility. Howell had thought of the Health Section of the League as a clearing house for information in regard to health conditions throughout the world, but it was aware that its influence was of a much more constructive and fundamental character.[53] In his answer to Howell, Russell emphasized that legal regulations in Europe laid down very definite requirements for the instruction and professional profile of the health officers and, according to his opinion, this had given rise to a more inflexible curriculum.

The policy of collaborative interaction and coordination between leaders of public health schools followed the same target as the program of interchange of public health officers, and meetings devoted to interchange of experiences between sanitary authorities were held also in other continents. In another chapter we shall discuss, for instance, the activities of the Singapore Bureau in the Far East. Furthermore, an international conference of Directors of African Health Administrations was also arranged by the Health Organization of the League at Entebbe, Lake Victoria, Uganda, particularly focused on strategies to cope with sleeping sickness.[54]

Generally speaking, the health authorities of most colonial administrations were anxious that the HO should continue its collaboration on African health problems in various directions such as the establishment of laboratories, boosting research on sleeping sickness and coordinating epidemiological research especially focused on the prevalence of tropical diseases. Similarly, the Health Committee was anxious to continue in this direction and, therefore, the approval of the HO was easily obtained. The Union of South Africa sent a request to organize a conference devoted to discuss public health problems as soon as possible. It was an urgent gathering of Chief Health Officers to discuss the prevention of yellow fever. The countries convened were the Union of South Africa, Southern Rhodesia, Northern Rhodesia, Portuguese East Africa, the Belgian Congo, French Equatorial Africa, Uganda, Tanganyika, Nigeria and possibly Kenya and India.

As a consequence of the 1930 Paris Conference and the enthusiastic coincidence of the positive effects of an international agreement on public health policies, the

French Government made a proposal for 'The Creation of an International School of Advanced Health Studies at Paris'.[55] The proposal discussed all the necessities, the technical organization, the teaching staff, number and type of students, general program of instruction, administrative organization and financial needs. The project was sent to the IHD of the Rockefeller Foundation after having been previously approved by the Council of the League of Nations. Bernard's report was accompanied by a letter of the French Government to the President of the Council of the League, and contained an annex entitled 'Organic Statutes of the International School of Advanced Health Studies'. Léon Bernard, as an expert and delegate of the French Government at the League, assumed the role of commentator. Rajchman demanded initially the opinion and agreement of the directors of national schools of public health, but there is no reference to such an agreement in the document.

When the Rockefeller Foundation received the proposal the IHD authorities requested the confidential opinion from a series of professors and experts in public health and also from Hampstead Laboratories and the Milbank Memorial Fund. Their response was unanimously positive towards the initiative and indeed the political process started when the Council of the League of Nations passed the proposal on 24 September 1930; the Health Section drew a draft informed by Léon Bernard, stating the commitment of the French Government with the creation of an International School of Advanced Health Studies with the support of the Rockefeller Foundation. The initiative was very ambitious. The international agents accepted the project, but seven years later, in 1937, the project was still not implemented. The parliamentary debate in France was not as easy as it had been at the international agencies. As a matter of fact the French Senate failed to commit the required funds. Again in 7 April 1938 the same story happened when the French Senate Financial Committee did not approve the details, the building or the allocation of funds and facilities. Finally, unfortunately it remained as a failed initiative because the ambitious project to create an international school of public health in Paris was never done.

On 29 June 1939 Rajchman visited the Rockefeller Foundation at New York together with Jean Monnet. Rajchman explained that the project of an international school of hygiene in Paris was finally stopped in the finances committee of the Senate of France. Caillaux, chairman of the finance committee and Ministry of Finance in France, was well disposed in favour of the initiative and the French Government could provide 1,000,000 French Francs for the maintenance, leaving the question of if the institution was to be located at Suresnes without a clear solution. An important detail is that the International School that Rajchman had in mind would not be intended for medical officers but for directors of schools of hygiene, a sort of coordinating institution. It would open six months a year with studies in the field and facilities from applying ideas in various fields. Rajchman thought of an international faculty, one group of which would serve from two to six months and another on a three-year appointment to develop some special field. A sum of 2,000,000 francs was estimated for the next two years to bring lecturers and provide scholarships for participants. A meaningful part of the funds were to be allocated by the participant governments.[56]

However, the war years introduced big changes in the Health Organization works and priorities. On 6 April 1942, a letter from S. Deutschman, former officer at the International Labour Office (ILO) and then in the United States, to George Strode, Associate Director IHD, RF stated:

> I have received a letter from Dr Biraud dated 16 February containing a paragraph which I think may interest you: En France une loi vient de créer à Paris un Institut National d'Hygiène sur le plan que vous connaissez; puisque c'est celui dejà envigé il y a un an. La direction en a été donnée par décret au Prof. André Chevallier, professeur de pharmacologie à Marseille, vu jadis avec le Dr Strode. Vous devinez ce que pense le Prof. Parisot qui a rejoint son post à Nancy.
>
> In France a law was recently passed to create a National Institute of Hygiene in Paris on the plans you know. It is the initiative already approved one year ago. The Decree appointed director Prof. Andrew Chevallier, Professor of Pharmacology at Marseille, formerly seen with Dr Strode. You guess what think Prof. Parisot who has returned to his post in Nancy.[57]

This was not the only unexpected news, because he also informed him that

> The Epidemiological Intelligence Service is carrying on its work in spite of the absence of data for the Far Eastern countries. The Singapore Branch has closed down on 20 January 1942, and Dr Park left for Australia. The Section is still receiving a number of requests for technical information from various health administrations. Dr Gautier and Dr Biraud recently wrote a short report on the nutrition situation in Europe intended for a study by Mr. Loveday at Princeton.[58]

Undoubtedly World War II changed the landscape radically and frustrated the international structure built during the previous decades by the League of Nations around public health.

The International Epidemiological Intelligence Service and Public Health Statistics

In addition to the instruction and interchange of public health officials, the coordination of schools of public health and the urgent fight against epidemics, famine and infectious diseases, a scheme to secure cooperation of the health administrations focused on the creation of an International Epidemiological Intelligence Service (IEIS) associated with an International Department of Public Health Statistics. It is easy to understand that any useful work in the field of health required a previous knowledge of the social and demographical context in order to assess the particularities and the extension of the health problems. This necessity was perceived in the course of the work undertaken by the Epidemics

Commission in Poland and Russia in the early 1920s. During this campaign, the efficacy of the preventive measures depended to a great extent upon the trustful information about the situation of the endemic places, the extension of the outbreaks and course of epidemics on both sides of the frontier. That is why the *European Health Conference* held in Warsaw in 1922 immediately claimed for the establishment of an International Epidemiological Intelligence Service, aiming to create epidemiological information available worldwide.

Prior to that initiative, during previous decades, many European Health Administrations at a series of International Conferences had struggled to secure an international exchange of epidemiological information. As said previously, the efforts culminated with the Rome agreement to establish the *Office International d'Hygiène Publique* in 1909 in Paris. The Office was supposed to collect and spread such epidemiological information and the conditions of public health settlements in different countries, but sometimes Governments were reluctant to circulate openly such an information or had no solid agencies to furnish trustful records, and when the Health Organization of the League entered the field, the *Office* was still publishing information which, as a matter of fact, was insufficient or useless for practical action.

At the International Sanitary Conference held in Warsaw in 1922, under the auspices of the League, a new principle was enunciated and then adopted: Health Administrations might communicate directly with each other and with the HO without intervention of Ministries of Foreign Affairs. When the Governments realized that no real harm resulted from the diffusion of those records, the volume of information circulating increased. On the other hand, the success of the HO in this field contributed to the improvement of the *Office International* system of collecting such information.[59]

On 27 May 1922 Wickliffe Rose confirmed that on 23 May the RF had approved the proposed scheme of cooperation for the creation of an IEIS for a five years period. On 14 June 1922

> the Executive Committee of the International Health Board, at his meeting on June 12, 1922, authorized the officers of the Board to enter into and arrangement with the Health Organization of the League of Nations for the maintenance of an epidemiological intelligence service on an international scale for a period of five years, beginning January 1, 1923, an for this purpose to commit the Board for assume not to exceed $32,840 for any one year.[60]

Just a few weeks later, on 3 July 1922 Ludwik Rajchman reported Rose all meetings and supports to the agreed program, and stated 'I am particularly anxious to say how glad I am of the impending close cooperation with the International Health Board and the intimate collaboration with Professor Selskar M. Gunn'.[61]

On 18 July 1922, L. Rajchman sent to Rose a personal letter enclosing the draft agreement and explaining to him that Manley O. Hudson, a member of the Legal Section of the Secretariat at the League and Professor of Civil Law at Harvard Law School had drafted the agreement for the scheme of both the Epidemiological Intelligence Service and the Interchange of Public Health Personnel.[62]

On 18 August the Agreement was approved. The RF introduced some minor corrections to the text and by 30 August Rajchman confirmed the acceptance of the corrections. Eric Drummond informed Rose that the Council of the League of Nations, at their meeting of 2 September 1922 had passed a Resolution inviting the Health Committee to consider the administration of the funds, placed by the Rockefeller Foundation, for the purpose of developing the Epidemiological Intelligence Service and instituting a program for the Interchange of Public Health Officials between various countries. Rose answered requesting to include the following description to Article 3 of the Agreement, where the aims of the program was described:

> a) Study of the simplest and most reliable methods of obtaining information regarding the incidence of disease and the progress of epidemics.
>
> b) Comparative study of public health statistics of different countries.
>
> c) Study of the world distribution of particular diseases.
>
> d) Comparative study of the incidence of particular diseases in different countries and their public health statistics, with a view to determining the nature and practical significance of observed difference between them.
>
> e) Study of the periodicity of epidemics and the factors, which cause or influence such periodicity.
>
> f) Organising, with the concurrence of the public health administrators of the countries affected, missions of enquiry regarding the development of epidemics.
>
> g) The publication and distribution of special reports and periodical bulletins.
>
> h) A review of the public health of the principal countries of the world with a view to the issue.
>
> i) Organising a rapid interchange of information in regard to particular diseases in cases in which immediate action appears to be necessary.
>
> j) The employment at headquarters or elsewhere of experts provided with requisite assistance and technical equipment.[63]

When the IEIS was established Europe was threatened by epidemics of cholera, typhus, dysentery and malaria from the Eastern countries and its first publications, the first three issues of the *Epidemiological Intelligence Bulletin* (January – June, 1922) were devoted to assess the importance of these problems.

From the very beginning Rajchman tried to convince Rose to involve the RF in the establishment of an IEIS and a Public Health Statistics Service. Indeed, on 23 May 1922 the Rockefeller Foundation approved the proposed scheme of cooperation for the International Epidemiological Intelligence Service proposed by the LNHO for a period of five years. On 14 June 1922 'the Executive Committee of the International Health Board, at his meeting on 12 June 1922, authorized the officers of the Board to enter into an arrangement with the LNHO for the maintenance of an epidemiological intelligence service on an international scale, based in Europe, for a period of five years, beginning 1 January 1923. For this purpose the RF IHB assumed not to exceed $32,840 per year.[64] Between 1922 and 1927, the RF contributed $350,000 to the LNHO for the program of institutionalization of vital statistics and epidemiological studies. On 18 July 1922, Rajchman issued Rose a personal letter enclosing the draft agreement and explaining to him that Manley O. Hudson, a member of the Legal Section of the Secretariat and Professor of Civil Law at Harvard Law School, had drafted the agreement for the scheme of the International Epidemiological Intelligence Service and Interchange of Public Health Personnel.

The only critical voice was that of George Buchanan, the British delegate, leading member of the *Office International d'Hygiène Publique* and vice-president of the Health Committee, who wrote a letter to Thorvald Madsen with a copy to Rajchman in which, regarding the International Epidemiological Intelligence Service and the Statistical Department, he claimed for a wider project involving the direction of the Health Organization, the *Office International d'Hygiène Publique* and 'in any case the action taken ought to be wholly under the responsibility and direction of the League, and not made a question for auxiliary funds'.[65] And he continued: 'In my view, it would be only seldom that there would be any advantage in undertaking these studies at Geneva. The conception of a super-epidemiologist at Geneva as pivot of the work seems to me radically unsound'.[66]

Buchanan's attitude was obstructive and contrary to the projects promoted by Rajchman in more than one case. In conclusion, Buchanan suggested that the Rockefeller IHB were invited to contribute a Rockefeller Fund for epidemiological intelligence and statistics, administered by the Health Committee primarily for the institution of those special comparative investigations of disease in different countries, which could be facilitated by utilizing the machinery of the Health Organization. The Health Committee should undertake this fact in the case that the annual sum suggested in the correspondence, i.e. 164,200 SF, was put at its disposal for this purpose. According to Buchanan, the fund should not be used, 'except perhaps in a minor way, for the appointment of salaried officers on the staff of the Health Section at Geneva'.[67]

Nevertheless, by the 18 August the Agreement was approved. The Rockefeller Foundation introduced some minor corrections and on 30 August Rajchman confirmed the acceptance of the corrections for the final version. Some of Buchanan's objections were not taken into consideration and the minutes of the International Health Board show that the 23 May the funds approved for the

IEIS were: 121,000 SF for salaries, publications and post expenses, and 285,200 SF per year for the period 1923–7 to attend the same concepts.

But the tension grew and Buchanan's criticism reached a higher political dimension. By August 1925 Mauden sent a letter to the Secretary General of the League of Nations and to the Assembly on the subjects of Mr Austen Chamberlain's remarks at the last meeting of the Council in which he criticized the Health Organization of the League. Selskar Gunn thought 'that the memorandum prepared by the Bureau of the Health Section answers quite effectively Mr Chamberlain's criticism. As I think I have already written to you, Mr Chamberlain was more or less an innocent mouthpiece in this case and the information, which he gave out was supplied by Sir George Buchanan. This, at any rate, is the version I have been given in the matter'.[68]

In undertaking the organization of the IEI Service on a worldwide scale the League was dependent upon national systems of vital statistics, a critical situation which could be supplemented in many complementary ways, but there was no substitute for national vital statistics regarding the supply of records. Moreover to be effective, information about health emergencies should be prompt and reliable and certainly only a few national systems for reporting diseases and deaths met both requirements in 1921.[69] The point of departure of the ambitious project was really deficient.

The argument insisted on the fact that the Health Section of the League created an IEI Service to meet the need of information on the health conditions of the populations, the epidemic outbreaks and the evolution of epidemics at any part of the world. As early as in 1921 the new service began to publish reports about the impaired health situation of many regions in Eastern Europe, drastically affected by typhus, relapsing fever and cholera, particularly in Russia and Poland, as a consequence of the post-war times. As we know, these previous efforts received the assistance and cooperation of the Soviet authorities. Undoubtedly the usefulness of epidemiological reports was essential for preventive strategies, to draft health policies and campaigns of intervention.

However, the position shown by the British representative, George Buchanan, was critical in several senses regarding the international epidemiology service project. As proof of that, he wrote to Thorvald Madsen on 27 July 1922 regarding the agreement signed with the RF and complaining about the British acceptation of some of the programs.[70] The letter was accompanied by a detailed report consisting of fifteen points related to the Rockefeller contributions that, on the other hand, he 'cordially welcome'.[71] Buchanan claimed that a separate fund distinct from the budget of the League, administrated apart and named 'Rockefeller Fund' should be created. He insisted on the fact that these funds were considered as auxiliary and not a part of the normal technical work, which the Health Organization had the duty of carrying out.

In practical terms he showed his opposition to the collaboration with the RF in this ambitious epidemiological project. What was the reason for his opposition to the project as conceived by the League and the Rockefeller leaders? Perhaps it was due to diplomatic reasons arising from its role as representative of the British government and the wish to safeguard the control of epidemiologic information. Or perhaps other institutional reasons derived from its leadership at the *Office Internationale d'Hygiene Publique*, which behind this initiative would surely lose much of its international role in the function of collecting international epidemiological information. Maybe the cause was personal feuds and disagreements with the leaders of the Health Organization. However that may be, Buchanan denied that there would be any advantage in undertaking that Service at Geneva. Obviously his obstructive attitude was commented on in confidential correspondence between the leaders of the LNHO and the RF.[72]

Notwithstanding the British distrust with the project, the Agreement was passed including some minor corrections and in November 1922, Gunn issued a copy of the 'Memorandum of the Medical Director to the Members of the Health Committee', focusing mainly on the initiation of the Epidemiology Intelligence Service.[73] Previously, the IHB of the RF at its meetings in May and October 1922, and at subsequent meetings of the Executive Committee, had discussed and approved a plan of cooperation with the LNHO providing for: a) aid toward the development of an epidemiological intelligence service to be conducted on an international scale; and b) aid in the development of a scheme of international exchange of sanitary personnel.

Once the project for the creation of an IEIS was approved, Rajchman requested support from the RF IHB in order to appoint the head of it, probably the most important piece to design and implement the service: 'If we are to establish our Epidemiological Intelligence Service on a really firm basis, and if you help us in this direction, we shall require the services of a first class epidemiologist and Public Health Statistician'.[74] On 6 May 1924, Gunn asked Russell, in the name of Rajchman, whether there was any possibility for the IHB taking on its regular staff Mr Sydenstricker and lending him to the League of Nations. Finally Edgar Sydenstricker, an expert of the USA Public Health Services, was appointed to organize and direct the Service for a period of at least two years.[75] Sydenstricker was a prominent public health statistician born in Shanghai, son of an American Presbyterian missionary, who had studied political economy at the University of Chicago and worked in the United States Public Health Service before being appointed by the League of Nations to lead the IEIS. Since 1921 he had started the Hagerstown Morbidity Survey in America following a similar approach of what was demanded for the new project of the League.[76]

In 1922 the epidemiological reports regarding the main infectious diseases were published periodically including all countries from east, west, north and south

Europe. With the international agreement about the list of infectious diseases of compulsory declaration (smallpox, malaria, diphtheria, dysentery, scarlet fever, tuberculosis, etc.) the reports of the IEI Service became more and more delayed and finally the first *Monthly Bulletin of Epidemiological Reports* (*Bulletin Mensuel de Renseignements Épidémiologiques*) of the Health Section was published in July 1923. The improvement of the service allowed this monthly updated information, which was available to national health authorities and other agencies working in national and international health. Just after the publication of the monthly reports, the first *Annual Epidemiological Report* (*Rapport Épidémiologique Annuel*) appeared as well in 1923, once the provisional records of the monthly reports were checked.

In 1923, after the Rockefeller Foundation had agreed to support the IEIS, the HO published some sort of comprehensive review of the prevalence of epidemic diseases in all European countries during 1922. By October of 1923, the IEIS was in a position to centralize the statistical returns of all European Health Administrations and to issue a carefully prepared comparative analysis of the situation in each country. The initial aim of the Epidemiological Service was simply to supply updated information to the authorities of European countries about the evolution of the health situation in neighbouring regions and countries. But with time passing, the importance of epidemiological data for social research and public health political action was soon recognized from several perspectives. The availability of comparable data allowed investigations about the geographical and the seasonal distribution of diseases, the comparison between countries and the rural and urban districts, giving the opportunity to assess the influence of climatic conditions, diet and many other factors.

Nevertheless the collection of records and the use of any statistical information required technical standardization to make information available and comparable. When trying to coordinate the information, epidemiologists and statisticians immediately recognized the difficulty to compare records from countries with an adequate statistical service with others where vital statistics and epidemiological records were simply non-existent, deficient or highly unsatisfactory. The standardization of the nomenclature of causes of death and statistical methods in epidemiology was essential for the development of the international health and for the expansion of social medicine. Therefore, a significant amount of work was made by the Health Organization to coordinate this target and make national statistical and epidemiological services more efficient as a way to facilitate the comparison of results. In this direction, the Epidemiological Intelligence Service played an essential role in the diffusion of statistical methods among different countries.[77] When it came to collect and publish morbidity and mortality statistics, the Geneva Epidemiological Intelligence Service realized that, for the purposes of comparison, it was absolutely necessary to standardize the methods of collecting and the statistical treatment of records. Statistical information required technical standardization to make it homologous and comparable.

Between 1923 and 1925 several Experts Committee meetings involving the heads of the epidemiological services in most European countries took place with the aim of planning a global report. Common rules to record causes of death were essential, but the project had to wait for a previous discussion on health care systems. Stillbirths was an outstanding case on which experts committees had succeeded in common agreements and most of the governments had adopted the same definition of the concept of *stillbirth* and a series of common rules for the compilation of statistics relating to it. This milestone allowed them to compare the figures furnished by health administration regarding birth rates, fertility rates and infant mortality rates. The international agreement introduced a change into demographic and health statistics, since after that the rates were calculated in relation to the number of *live* births and not to the *total* births.[78]

As a consequence of the agreement, soon information was received in Geneva from most of the well-organized epidemiological services and health administrations in the world, which had records available or could easily obtain them, and the publications of the League stimulated health administrations to improve their own services. Only countries without a fair system of data collection failed to make returns to the League, and these related particularly to China and some other Asiatic countries and a number of Central and Latin American countries. Africa was, in fact, a colonial territory. A step forward was taken by the Health Committee in February 1924 when it was decided to appoint special committees of statisticians to survey certification of causes of death and methods of classifying them, when more than one cause is given. International homologation required uniformity in the statistical presentation of mortality records with special reference to sex and age groups, as well as a clear definition of stillbirths and the agreement on population standards for use in the mortality rates. The first committee to complete its work was the one dealing with the definition of stillbirths. After long debates and negotiations an agreed definition was adopted; twenty-two countries expressed agreement; Australia, Brazil and South-Africa stated that they were to introduce new regulations. However the British Government was unable to adopt the definition proposed and as a consequence of its criticism a new, more flexible method was adopted. Countries in which a different definition was in legal use were asked to tabulate infant mortality in two ways, first according to the national, and second according to the international definition. This solution was accepted by the British Registrars and agreed with other critical countries, which had shown previous criticism, and finally a reasonable degree of international uniformity was secured. In October to December 1924 a 'Provisional Outline of Topics for Collective Study of Vital Statistics' was produced, as organized by the Health Section of the League of Nations.[79]

It included the discussion of general methods and procedures for the collecting and statistical treatment of data regarding special diseases such as tuberculosis, malaria, venereal diseases, puerperal sepsis, diphtheria and occupational diseases. The next target was the decennial revision of the International List of Causes of Death. The Health Committee undertook preparatory work in 1925 setting up a committee to discuss several options and lists of causes of death that were circulated to Governments. In 1929 a joint committee of the Health Committee with the French International Institute of Statistics was created to prepare an agreed report for the Conference. The List of Causes of Death, which issued from the Conference, was assured of good reception and the Health Organization ensured a considerable advance in the international comparability of vital and health statistics.[80] The next step was uniformity in the presentation of morbidity statistics.A specific program for training officials in the service of various Governments in order to improve vital and health statistics was approved by the Council of the League on 7 July 1923. The importance of this training was based on the need for introducing similar methods in the statistical practices of most countries bringing into closer contact medical statisticians of various countries.[81] This project was in fact an outgrowth of the establishment of the International Epidemiological Intelligence Service and Public Health Statistics and followed similar patterns and principles as the program for interchange of public health personnel. For this program the RF made available 10,500 SF in 1923 and 21,000 SF yearly from 1924 to 1927. The first use of the grant was to organize a group of medical statisticians and epidemiologists for the study of vital statistics at the central headquarters of the League in Geneva, as well as in other cities in Switzerland, Paris, The Hague and London. Participants were elected by the health administration of eight countries. After spending six weeks in Geneva devoting most of the time to the study of vital statistics and the epidemiological work of the League, they paid visits to statistical agencies in the above-mentioned cities, and the program ended with a series of final conferences in Geneva. Those interchanges started in 1923 and were repeated during the following years with an increasing number of participants and visits to a wider range of statistical offices in Denmark, Sweden, Norway, Scotland, England and other countries.

On 30 May 1924, when the ambitious international collection of data started, Eichel issued a letter to Russell stating that many countries did not issue any information at all for the monthly epidemiological reports. 'Probably the largest and most important missing is China'. Only records from Hong Kong were available. 'The same consideration as above apply to Central and South America ... Bolivia, Chile, Colombia, Guatemala, Panamá Republic, Paraguay, Venezuela, Nicaragua'.[82]

Mr Sydenstricker made previous diplomatic attempts to get in contact with officials in these countries, but he never received replies to his communications, possibly because in some or all of these countries there was no central statistical Bureau or a similar agency able to provide such information.[83]

On 20 June 1924, Florence M. Read answered to Eichel's 30 May previous letter. Russell was at that time absent of the Office on a working tour in Japan:

> With reference to China, Mr Roger S. Greene, Director of the China Medical Board of the Rockefeller Foundation, wrote to Mr Sydenstricker under date of March 10, 1924, concerning possible sources of epidemiological information for China ... The Board's representative in China is Dr John B. Grant, who is at present serving as Associate Professor of Hygiene and Public Health at Peking Union Medical College ... In Central and South America we have the following representatives: Guatemala: Dr John E. Elmerdorf, Jr; Nicaragua: Dr D.M. Molloy; Panama: Dr Louis Schapiro; Paraguay: Dr Fred L. Soper. In Colombia the suggested contact was Pablo García Medina (Director Nacional de Higiene) and Juan N. Corpas (Cabinet Ministro Instrucción y Salubridad Públicas).[84]

In addition to the funds, archival documents show that the Rockefeller international network and diplomatic contacts played an important role in the development of this project. However, apparently the RF had no representatives in Bolivia, Chile and Venezuela.

On 15 April 1924, Russell wrote to Gunn:

> It seems to me that the Division of Epidemiological Intelligence has been developed by Mr Sydenstricker to such an extent, that it is already fairly well established, and it still has nearly four years to run before our appropriations cease. In other words, it seems to me that the chances are that this Division which we have helped to establish will be taken over at the end of the preliminary period by the League of Nations.[85]

Regarding vital statistics the Rockefeller leaders considered that temporary activities might arise in the future and it did not seem essential that the League should continue this activity. A program of study tours took them to Switzerland, France the Netherlands and the three Scandinavian countries, where those experts were aware of the advantages of coordinating and standardizing statistical methods and, where necessary, to improve the traditional way of doing things in their own countries.

On 2 September 1924, Gunn informed Russell about the approval of the proposal for a Bureau of Epidemiological Intelligence for the Far East shaped and developed under the leadership of the League.[86] Rajchman had previously issued a report to Gunn[87] about the Service of Epidemiological Intelligence, Official statistical records:

> During the autumn of 1923 a group of 9 officials, representing as many countries, were brought together for a period of several months to study collectively the problems of official vital statistics and the methods of several important offices ... During the present year there have been in progress special studies on cerebrospinal meningitis, by Dr Seligmann of Berlin; on scarlet fever and diphtheria by Dr Rosenfeld of Vienna. This research has for its object the elucidation of some of the important factors which

> influence the statistics of these diseases and which may affect their international comparability ... Further, The Service of Epidemiological Intelligence was visited at Geneva, upon its invitation, by the following experts, for personal conferences and statistical problems: Professor Niceforo of Italy, Monsieur Ney of Switzerland, Dr Rosenfeld of Austria, Dr Roesle of Prussia, Dr Würzburger of Saxony and Dr Hansen of Denmark. The Service also confered with Dr Wroczynski of Poland on the technical aspects of proposed legislation for registration of deaths.[88]

Rajchman announced the submission to the Health Committee of the League of a proposal for a world registration area for notifiable diseases. The working group appointed to discuss a proposal on standardization of Causes of Death was composed by: Stevenson (England), Davis (USA), Rosenfeld (Austria) and Roesle (Germany). Another on Standard Million Population was composed by Niceforo (Italy), Würzburger (Saxony), Wilson (USA) and Brownlee (England). A third was devoted to Age & Sex Classification of Causes of Death composed by Hansen (Denmark), Coats (Canada), Pearl (USA) and Aschieri (Italy). The Joint Committee on Still Births was integrated by Dudfield (England), Huber (France), Eardley Holland (England), Ney (Switzerland) and Hedren (Sweden).

In a report dated the 8 September 1924, Rajchman informed Gunn that the staff engaged in the Epidemiological Service was paid using funds from the League (30,000 SF). Publications amounted 43,750 SF for 1924 and 60,000 for 1925. Some special reports, enquiries and technical investigations made a total amount of 162,000 SF. All travelling expenses were assumed by the League of Nations.[89] On 19 September 1924 Russell confirmed with Gunn the RF commitment of $50,000 for the first year and $125,000 for the next five-year period. This scheme shows the involvement of both institutions for the consolidation of the international standardization of causes of death.

At the 1925 meeting, the epidemiology group of experts agreed to draw up a number of common rules relating to the registration of the causes of death. Special emphasis was laid on the necessity for introducing medical data of the death certificates in the civil register, safeguarding professional secrecy and privacy, as something essential for the certificates to be reliable. This committee of experts played an important part, together with the International Statistical Institute, in the preparation of the agenda for the decennial revision of the International List of Causes of Death, which took place in 1929.

Although statistics could be standardized by a simple agreement between statisticians and medical experts in the various countries, in practical terms considerable difficulties arose due to a deficient demographic and epidemiologic system of recording records in many countries, together with local traditions, national legislations and political decisions. Both the League of Nations and the Rockefeller Foundation were pioneering standardization projects in many aspects related to health and medical practice. The point of departure was chaotic due to the heterogeneity of situations. The documents that had been compiled during decades were conceived according to rules, which varied widely among countries. This made difficult comparability and therefore the Committee of Experts prepared guidelines in collecting demographic and epidemiologic data, something that made it possible to interpret the statistics of some twenty countries without hard research in libraries.

Rajchman expressed this idea in all his public interventions and writings defending international standardization strategies, but once more the international initiatives were seen sometimes as foreign intrusion into national matters. This was the case of George Buchanan, the British representative, often suspicious and critical with the HO decisions and with the internationalization of certain public health strategies. In spite of the positive availability of comparable records in different countries, Buchanan mistrusted the internationalist perspective of the experts and their wish to influence national policies and what he considered as pure domestic affairs. Great Britain initially turned down the initiative of a series on *International Health Yearbooks.*

Despite the initial controversy, an *International Health Yearbook* was finally published in 1925 with the direct collaboration of twenty-two countries. Rajchman sent a letter to the national authorities requesting updated reports on demographic and epidemiologic records, sanitary reforms, public health policies and detailed information about social diseases. The *International Health Yearbook* was published for five years, 1925–30, and included valuable records on the international health situation by the International Labour Office (ILO), the International Red Cross and the RF. The number of participants grew from year to year and thirty-seven countries participated, sending their records and sanitary information in 1929. However, inevitable deficiencies in the technical coordination and in methodological and linguistic standardization made the final results a bit disappointing and heterogeneous. After the 1929 crash the situation worsened and funds from the RF shrank. Finally, the 1930 issue was the last one issued. The deep depression affected seriously the continuity of the program.

Nevertheless the *International Health Yearbook* had serious limitations. It simply summarized and compiled national reports without any hope on comparative transnational analysis or conclusive criticism. A scrupulous respect to keep away from suspicious of any *internal affairs* prevented from going forward of this purely descriptive and non-intrusive approach to the social meaning of epidemiological records. International diplomacy and political tensions were at a critical moment and any sort of criticism could be misinterpreted by national political authorities. Reports contained in the yearbook offered demographic and epidemiologic records and information about institutions, facilities, sanitary staff, health care, health insurances and other topics regarding public health organization. One of its main contributions was the establishment of a real network of circulating international information, available to national governments and public health experts, as a tool to plan health policies, reinforcing the necessity of national offices for vital statistics as an instrument for decisions making. Campaigns against malaria and other infectious diseases, surveys on health status of the population as well as nutrition deficiencies in rural areas were mainly identified according to the establishment of epidemiologic information. Since 1929, the *Monthly Epidemiological Reports* also included enquiries and a wide bibliography about the most important infectious diseases and other health problems and health care initiatives considered of interest at any moment. Monographic surveys on specific topics were published as well about diphtheria, smallpox, scarlet fever, tularemia, typhus, psittacosis and infant paralysis. However the big economic and financial crash in 1930 and their consequences for unemployment and for the impairment of social wellbeing ended up with this ambitious program of expert circulating information. Indeed the standardization of morbidity statistics was still a remaining field of agreement for the activities of the Committee of Experts Statisticians. Some progress was gained early in the 1920s with the agreement on compulsory notification of a list of contagious diseases. The problem became more complex and hard to solve when an attempt was made to draw up a list of diseases requiring special needs and social insurance. No previous list like the one, that had been internationally agreed for a classification of diseases, included diseases causing some sort of working incapacity. Therefore, the most important insurance companies in the different countries used lists, which often lacked any medical background and seldom were of any great value. This was a hot point in health politics. At the same time, certain social groups such as workers' unions and political movements tried to influence and modify the predominant statistical and technological orientation of social medicine promoted by the RF and LNHO, highlighting the importance of civil rights and calling for more attention to women's health, housing, workers' health, control of natality and similar issues as important topics to be included in the agenda, but these initiatives had in fact little effect on data-collecting policies. The Health Committee of the League, in common with the RF's International Health Board/ Division, was more concerned with the instruction of public health experts and promoting a technical approach to the diagnosis and treatment of health problems even considering their social dimension. As a result of the work done, the Health Organization published a series of volumes on public health services, organization and working activities of the following countries: Australia, Austria, Belgium, Bulgaria, Czechoslovakia, Denmark, France, French colonies, Germany, Hungary, British India, Italy, Japan, Latvia, the Netherlands, New Zealand, Norway, Poland, Ukraine and Yugoslavia. A series of statistical handbooks on the statistical methods used and the statistical data available in Austria, Belgium, Canada, Czechoslovakia, England and Wales, France, Hungary, Irish

Free State, Northern Ireland, the Netherlands, Portugal, Scandinavia, Scotland, Spain and Switzerland, and six volumes of the *International Health Yearbook* contained reports regarding at least twenty-two countries.[90] All these publications contained a huge amount of information that probably was not directly useful for practical purposes, but showed the importance of the internationalization movement. The continuity of the Epidemiological Service and its programs were assured until the Rockefeller Foundation engagement was extinguished at the end of 1934. After the end of this period of collaboration, the ambitious international epidemiology program was to be carried on exclusively by the League of Nations. In 1930 the staff of the Service consisted of a chief, a statistician, a technical member of the Section, one secretary typist, seven clerks and a draughtsman. Should the support of the RF cease at the end of 1934, the Chief of the Service would not have his contract renewed and four clerks would have to leave, losing leadership and capacity of action for new planning and enterprises.

The Eastern Epidemiological Bureau at Singapore

The evident usefulness of the International Epidemiological Service and its immediate recognized success prompted the Japanese member of the Health Committee, soon after its creation in 1922, to request the Health Organization to examine the epidemiological conditions in the Far East and to consider the possibility of establishing in the Asian region a similar service to the one created in Geneva. A member of the Epidemics Commission made a formal request and this was the starting point of the Eastern Epidemiological Intelligence Bureau based in Singapore. In the election of the site the most important thing was the central position and exceptional dimension and importance of Singapore's port for the whole maritime trade between Japan, China, the Near East, Africa and Europe. To prepare such an ambitious project, a conference of the representatives of the Far-Eastern Health Administrations was held in Singapore in February 1925. It approved the establishment of the Epidemiological Bureau, which became operative just a few weeks later.[91]

On 17 June 1923, the Medical Director Ludwik Rajchman was authorized by a resolution of the Council to enter into formal negotiations with the RF regarding the support of a Bureau of Epidemiological Intelligence at Singapore and finally the agreement was signed in 1924. On 20 May 1924 minutes of the International Health Board of the Rockefeller Foundation say that a proposal from the Health Committee of the League had been received asking for aid to establish an Epidemiological Intelligence Bureau in the Far East. It was presented to the LN Health Committee in February 1924 and Rajchman submitted a request to the Rockefeller Foundation through Selskar Gunn on 12 March 1924. As a positive answer, the IHB of the Rockefeller Foundation

> resolved that the cooperation of the Boarding the establishment of an EPIDEMIOLOGICAL INTELLIGENCE BUREAU of the League of Nations in the FAR EAST as outlined above be, and it is hereby, approved in principle ... committing the Board in a sum not to exceed $50,000 for the first year and not to exceed $125,000 for a five-year period.[92]

The initial agreements were active until 1927. A summary of the funds assigned were as follows:

	RF Funds	**Total Budget HO**
	In Swiss Francs	
1922	132,300 ($25,540)	392,125 ($75,699)
1923	153,200 (29,274)	700,500 (135,231)
1924	191,250 (37,112)	641,120 (123,768)
1925	238,925 (46,126)	809,764 (156,325)
1926	257,460 (49,702)	988,165 (190,765)
1927	385,527 (74,425)	991,115 (191,335)

Table 3.2: **(1) Grant by the Rockefeller Foundation for the Far East Epidemiological Bureau of the Health Organization at Singapore.**

For the next five years the schedule was progressively reduced as follows, according to the 1927 prevision:

1928:	$50,000
1929:	$45,000
1930:	$40,000
1931:	$35,000
1932:	$30,000

Table 3.3: **(2) Grant by the Rockefeller Foundation for the Far East Epidemiological Bureau of the Health Organization at Singapore.**

In March 1928 it was agreed to combine pledges for the Epidemiological Intelligence Service and the establishment of a centre of public health documentation:

1928:	$60,335
1929:	$48,995
1930:	$44,155
1931:	$39,315
1932:	$34,475
1933:	$29,635
1934:	$22,400

Table 3.4: **(3) Grant by the Rockefeller Foundation for the Far East Epidemiological Bureau of the Health Organization at Singapore.**

For the Epidemiological Intelligence Bureau of the Far East (agreement 1924 expiring 1929) the total amount estimated not to exceed $125,000 over the five-year period.

Epidemiological Intelligence:

1923	$40,340
1924	$53,840
1925	$53,840
1926	$53,840
1927	$53,840
1928	$50,000
1929	$45,000
Total	$350,700

Table 3.5: **(4) Grant by the Rockefeller Foundation for the Far East Epidemiological Bureau of the Health Organization at Singapore.**

International Interchange of Public Health Personnel

1922	$15,020
1923	$63,080
1924	$80,040
1925	$100,000
1926	$75,000
1927	$66,224
1928	$51,515
1929	$50,000
Total	$500,880

Table 3.6: **(5) Grant by the Rockefeller Foundation for the Far East Epidemiological Bureau of the Health Organization at Singapore.**

In 1935 the total amount was $100,000.

In accordance with the agreement, the functions of the Epidemiological Intelligence Bureau in the Far East were summarized in the following six issues:

1. To collect and transmit at regular intervals, from all Far Eastern countries, information regarding the incidence and spread of infectious diseases, especially in ports and their hinterland.
2. To collect and transmit periodical returns of vital statistics in Far East ports.
3. To collect data regarding alterations, additions or amendments to sanitary laws and regulations, and regarding measures taken to combat transmissible diseases and to prevent their propagation.
4. To publish at regular intervals, returns, data, tables and general vital statistics regarding Far Eastern countries.
5. To transmit all the above-mentioned information periodically to the ports and health administrations of all the Far Eastern countries concerned, and also to the Health Section of the League of Nations, whose duty it shall be to communicate them to the *Office International*

d'Hygiène Publique and to the various national health administrations.

6 To render all possible assistance to the Governments concerned in matter which fall within its competence.[93]

The Rockefeller Foundation appropriated for this purpose the sum of 125,000 SF to be spread over a period of five years starting in 1925.[94] Grants received by the HO from the RF subsequent to 1929, in view of the consolidated grant agreement, were utilized in part for the support of the Bureau.

From a global perspective, social diseases affecting different regions showed very plural situations in a time of political and economic instability and epidemiological transitions. In Europe, pest and cholera were rare and, only in Russia, those traditional epidemics had gained ground as a consequence of the negative post-war conditions, the economic crisis and the social instability, provoking an impairment of the living conditions among the lowest social groups. On the contrary, these diseases were always prevalent as an endemic problem in China, India and other Eastern countries making the affected regions an obstacle for the commercial interest of the big powers and dangerous sources of contagion to their neighbours, as well as a real threat for the free circulation of ships. Quarantine measures and maritime traffic regulations were very important in this context and the reaction of governments was very strict particularly after the transmission of pest into Java and the outbreaks of cholera in Japan during the years prior to the agreement. Eastern authorities were concerned with trying to regulate and improve the efficiency of quarantines and called for information and surveillance, cooperating very proactively with the activities of the new Asian Epidemiologic Bureau. As soon as it was established, they supplied the requested information and gave subsidies for the best functioning and the immediate circulation of the available information.

As soon as the preparatory work had been carried out, including visits to the most important ports in the area, a Regional Conference gathering the health authorities concerned was called in Singapore in February 1925. Prior to that, Thorvald Madsen met the RF leaders in New York in October 1924 to arrange financial details, and finally the RF contributed $5,000 for organization expenses and for the travel of the public health expert Norman White – the British senior official of the LNHO with experience in health problems in Asia – while the rest of the Eastern participants assumed their own expenses.[95]

In a confidential report, Norman White wrote to F. F. Russell around the International Conference to be held in Singapore:

> the sum of $50,000 is an outside estimate of the cost of one year's working of the bureau even when fully established; it may be considerably less. The administrations directly interested in the matter are: Straits Settlements, Federated Malay States, Dutch East Indies, Siam, French Indo-China, Australia, Hong Kong, China, Shanghai and other Chinese Treaty Ports, Japan, Korea and South Manchuria Railway Administration, the Philippine Islands, British India, Ceylon, Russian Maritime Province, and Portuguese Colonies.[96]

The European powers had a pure colonial interest. Norman White proposed a meeting with the delegates of the countries on 25 February 1925 and considered a sum of $40,000 to be sufficient to install the bureau and maintain the first year of work. Therefore, the plan for the installation and working of an Epidemiological Intelligence Bureau for the Far East in Singapore was adopted, including an Epidemiological Intelligence Service, which also assumed other functions such as collecting records, regulations and laws, measures taken to fight infectious diseases, publication of statistics and assistance to governments.

By the 13 March 1924 the working program was approved[97] and by the 8 December 1924 an agreement between the LN and the Rockefeller Foundation, on behalf of its International Health Board for the Establishment and Maintenance of the Epidemiological Intelligence Bureau in the Far East, was also approved. The IHB agreed to pay an initial grant of $50,000 and $125,000 for the next five year period.[98]

The Singapore Conference officially approved the establishment of the Bureau, defined the above-mentioned functions and established a preliminary list of the ports with which the epidemiological program would be concerned. Several Governments agreed to make contributions towards its upkeep and two of them offered to place their wireless stations at the Bureau's disposal for broadcasting the weekly information. Within a few months after its establishment, practically all the health administrations in the area were sending weekly telegrams reporting the situation of their ports regarding epidemic and contagious diseases.[99]

The Bureau started working in late February 1925 and its first telegram was received on 25 February from Hong Kong. Twelve countries represented at the Conference agreed to furnish weekly telegraphic returns from thirty-five ports.[100] Incoming telegrams notified the Bureau of the first appearance of cholera, human or rat plague, smallpox, yellow fever or unusual prevalence rates or mortality rates from any infectious disease. Regular weekly telegrams gave for important ports numbers of cases and deaths from any unusual epidemic outbreaks. This information was made into a bulletin and telegraphed in a special code to all the health administrations in the area, which extended from Africa in the West, to Vladivostok in the East.

On 14 February 1925 Rajchman showed his satisfaction to Gunn: 'You will be glad to know that the Singapore Conference has proved a very great success. The following administrations were represented: British North Borneo, Ceylon, China, Dutch East Indies, Federated Malay States, French Indochina, Hong Kong, India, Japan, Philippine Islands, Straits Settlements. Proceedings started on 4 February and finished the 13th'.[101]

A couple of years later, in 1927, Heiser sent to the RF authorities a memorandum on the International Conference on South Pacific Health Problems, a meeting held in Australia. The report covered the absence of any delegate from the USA attending the Conference.

> Great Britain sent Sir George Buchanan, and all the various British countries sent delegates, including New Zealand, Samoa, Cook Islands, Fiji, etc. Dr Norman White, from whom this statement was obtained, was sent by the League of Nations. According to N. White, Sir George Buchanan continued his insidious attacks on the League, and White felt that while very little of a constructive nature was accomplished by the Australian conference, his presence could be justified on the ground of blocking destructive measures that Sir George might have brought about. There was no discussion of the plan of the IHB to cooperate with the High-Commission group.[102]

On 14 March 1927 the Singapore Bureau had prioritized the following program of topics to challenge immediately:

a) Chlorinization of water.
b) Fumigation of ships.
c) Survey on quarantine procedures applied in the Far East countries.
d) Investigations around storage of grain.
e) Rat survey in the ports.
f) Preventive inoculation of cholera vaccine, buccal vaccine and others.
g) Studies of selected centres of cholera and plague.
h) Special Interchange initiatives among Port Health Officers of the Far East Network.
i) Assistance in training subsidiary personnel in native states.
j) Training of Chinese officials taking over sanitary administration of areas previously in the hands of Europeans.

Although the decade of the 1930s was very critical for coordinated international public health action in many senses, the 1931 evaluation report circulated among the Rockefeller authorities showed a very optimistic assessment of the Far East Epidemiological Service: 'Thus for the first time an international epidemiological service had been established capable of collecting and transmitting with the speed demanded by the requirements of modern transportation, current information on the prevalence of epidemic diseases in the ports most subject to such infection'.[103] The weekly information sent each Wednesday from Singapore by telegraph and wireless related to the week ending the previous Saturday midnight. At the end of 1925 the work of the Bureau was extended to sixty-five ports, and a weekly fasciculus containing additional information about the prevalence of diseases in ports and countries, quarantine measures, meteorology and other valuable information was also published.

The Bureau informed the Governments of the region about the appearance of epidemics in certain ports and thus they could immediately adopt the necessary preventive measures of protection against ships coming from those contaminated ports. At the same time, local authorities could know as well that they could dispense all the ships from non-infected areas. The Bureau information had the double advantage of increasing security and eliminating unnecessary quarantine restrictions on maritime trade. In accordance with this practical dimension, the information and services of the Eastern Bureau became really most effective if they covered the widest possible area. To reach this goal, along the huge region bounded on the east by Panama, on the north by Vladivostok and on the west by Suez, the Bureau established initially weekly telegraphic communication with thirty-five ports, and one decade later the information framework had increased spectacularly, applying to one hundred and fifty maritime stations. The Epidemiological Intelligence Service covered, in 1931, all Eastern ports of any importance except some Chinese ports due to political disturbances.

The ports informed the Singapore Bureau telegraphically about the number of cases and deaths caused by epidemic diseases every week and even more often when necessary. The health administrations notified as well of the establishment or removal of quarantine measures and, in some instances, of the departure and the itinerary followed by infected boats. Ports situated near an area affected by an epidemic outbreak were notified by telegram in urgent cases and they could indeed take preventive measures in time. The Bureau summarized the information received from all points of the Pacific in a *Bulletin*, which was sent weekly by telegraph in a special code to the Geneva Epidemiological Centre and to the Health Authorities of the Eastern countries. The authorities in Indochina, the Netherlands' Indies, British India, Madagascar, China, Japan and Germany placed their stations at the disposal of the Eastern Bureau for the purpose of reducing costs and facilitating the dissemination of information over a wider territory. Arrangements were made to broadcast the weekly bulletin reports in code from a number of stations. Starting in 1930, the Bureau was able to issue daily information through the Malabar station in Java on a wavelength of 600 metres so that the messages could be picked up at sea. The weekly broadcasting of epidemiological information issued by the Eastern Epidemiological Bureau was ensured daily in 1931 by ten stations and one station broadcast. The epidemiological centre of Melbourne also sent to the Bureau information from the Southern Pacific archipelagos and the *Conseil Sanitaire Maritime et Quarentenaire* in Egypt who were informed about epidemics and outbreaks of any contagious disease among the pilgrims going to Hedjaz, west of present Saudi Arabia. Those records were highly important for Muslim countries. As we have discussed in a previous chapter, this complex network was the result of decades of sanitary international diplomacy, started in the mid-nineteenth century with the International Sanitary Conferences.

When the International Sanitary Convention entered into force in 1926, the Eastern Epidemiology Intelligence Bureau acted as intermediary between the health authorities in Asia and the *Office International d'Hygiène Publique*. A double function characterized the Singapore Bureau. On the one hand, it notified the health authorities of the movements of infected ships and the evolution of epidemiological records; on the other, the Bureau contributed to inform about the most effective methods of disinfection and quarantine. The Bureau collected and distributed information on the health facilities in the port stations and some public health experts from different countries visited and exchanged experiences to promote valuable cooperation between directors of maritime sanitary stations. With the target of improving public health measures the Health Committee of the League of Nations set up a Commission of Enquiry into the Fumigation of Ships and obtained the close cooperation of the United States Federal Health Service.

The Eastern Bureau developed an advisory role acting as an intermediary between the health administrations and governments in the region. Governments sent delegates to the yearly sessions of its Advisory Council, which took place in different cities such as Singapore, New Delhi, Bandung and others. The delegates exchanged information and points of view, and assessed the sanitary situation in the wide region. Therefore, not only the technical dimension of its works was considered to be important, the Bureau also developed a very extensive diplomatic activity in the processes of negotiation health policies. In one of the Council meetings, authorities requested the Bureau to undertake investigations into the efficacy of oral vaccinations against cholera and dysentery and, as a consequence, the Bureau stimulated research on this particular topic.

The topic had a certain tradition. Valuable research had been done in British, Portuguese and French India, in Siam, and other places. Oral vaccination against cholera was proved experimentally in Madras and the results were assessed as being equally effective as the previous campaigns using subcutaneous vaccination. The Eastern Bureau obtained similar results with the testing of anti-dysentery bacteriophage and with dried anti-smallpox vaccine. The international experts considered the efficacy being greatly superior to the vaccinal lymph normally used in tropical countries and on board ships. All this research on cholera was carried out on behalf of the Singapore Bureau. A valuable report on this subject was prepared by Colonel Russell of India and published at the central headquarters of the League in Geneva summarizing the results. A number of administrations undertook carrying out experiments in oral vaccination against cholera and dysentery in Portuguese India, Pondicherry, Cochin China, Singapore, Sumatra, Sian and British India.[104]

As an international agency, the Bureau acted as well as a coordinator for research into plague. It assumed this role after a meeting of the committee of experts held in Calcutta in 1927. The work was distributed amongst the different services and laboratories in the area and then the health authorities exchanged the results obtained through the Bureau, which convened periodical meetings. Research about plague, according to the program elaborated by the Bureau, was started in Siam, Hong Kong, Indo-China, Union of South Africa, Australia, Ceylon and the Netherlands East Indies. Following with this task of intermediation, the Bureau likewise acted between a large number of laboratories in the

East and Far East for the exchange of information, use of experimental animals, production of vaccines, bacterial strains and laboratory research facilities.[105]

With the time passing, the Eastern Bureau in Singapore became something other than a simple office for the exchange of epidemiological intelligence records. It developed an active role in regional public health policies oriented by the League, as well a diplomatic function connecting links between health authorities in this wide region and assumed demands from the governments and experts to coordinate likewise experimental research. Indeed it played a meaningful role in the program of expansion of Western medicine in China, boosted by the Rockefeller Foundation and other American institutions, and then supported by the League and by other medical and philanthropic institutions.

On March 1928 Rajchman initiated conversations with G. K. Strode and Russell in order to guarantee the continuity of the activities of the Eastern Bureau at Singapore with the aid of the Rockefeller Foundation.[106] He remembered that the Eastern Bureau was founded initially to act as a branch office of the International Epidemiological Intelligence Service with site in Geneva and that the IHD Rockefeller grant was initially made available for a five years period ending on 31 December 1929. Meanwhile, the Bureau received financial contributions from certain Far Eastern Administrations and from the League, which had already assumed the maintenance of the Bureau as an official centre of epidemiological intelligence in the frame of their own institutions. However, Rajchman insisted on its consideration that the Bureau had evolved into a general agency for the countries in the Far East for all activities related to international health.

In addition to research to give impulse to oral vaccination and epidemiological enquiries about cholera and plague, the authorities of the Bureau had established contact with health administrations of most Asian countries. A survey was circulated to coordinate study programs among public health services and national health institutes in the semi-autonomous states and colonial possessions and territories in regard to serum-diagnosis methods for syphilis, in the standardization of biological products, prevention and treatment of malaria, control of infant mortality and some aspects of sanitary engineering to improve health care facilities. The Advisory Board of the Bureau drew up at its 1928 session, a comprehensive program of epidemiological and laboratory studies and surveys on the dimension of plague and a survey on the consequences of quarantine measures in Far East ports.[107]

The Advisory Council had been established in 1926 and was made up of representatives of the health administrations from the Netherlands, East Indies, French Indo-China, British Colonies, British India, Japan and Japanese Colonies, Siam, China and the Observer of the Philippines. The presence and influence of experts coming from the Western empires were predominant and the main forces for the coordination and implementation of public health policies. This council met yearly, passed upon the report of the Director, approved the budget and made suggestions for future plans and recommendations for national policies. Soon after its establishment the Advisory Council suggested that the Singapore Bureau should take up a number of subjects of particular interest: malaria research, oral vaccination against acute intestinal infections, endemic foci of cholera, rat and flea habitat, pneumonia plague and tuberculosis.[108]

In connection to this, repeated demands were presented by members of the Health Committee for the organization of a program of interchanges for health officers acting in maritime sanitary stations in the Far Eastern area and for facilities to be given for individual studies by selected port officers in regard to fumigation of ships, spread of plague through defective grain storage and collaboration between port authorities of different countries regarding the transit of infected ships, among other more simple or particular issues. Those activities were not included in the scope of the arrangement made in 1925 between the HO and the RF, and therefore Rajchman asked if the IHD of the RF would be prepared to conclude a new agreement to enable the Bureau to fulfil new functions for a longer period of seven years. The program proposed by Rajchman included the following issues:

1. Investigation and evaluation of the effectiveness of quarantine in Far East ports.
2. Study of the best methods of fumigation of ships in freight.
3. Study of the plague spread in regard to defective grain storage and measures to be taken to improve the situation.
4. Uniform strategies for rat and flea control in the ports.
5. Interchanges and individual missions for health officers to share experiences.
6. Epidemic outbreaks and fight against cholera in different areas.
7. Study of the factors responsible for the disappearance of plague in certain ports like Hong Kong.
8. Assessment of preventive vaccination against cholera, plague and dysentery: oral vaccines, ingestion of bacteriophage, subcutaneous inoculation.
9. Extension of the work of the Malaria Commission to training of experts, application of anti-mosquito and anti-larval measures, coordination of studies at the Institutes of Hygiene in the Far East countries.
10. Discussion about the best methods for chlorination of drinking water.
11. Cooperation with health administrations for training auxiliary sanitary staff, particularly at Siam, India and independent countries of the Far East region.
12. Collaboration through technical advice with the Chinese Health Service.

When Rajchman sent the proposal to the IHD of the RF the facilities and staff of the Singapore Bureau could not assume and develop by their own means any aspect of this ambitious program. A selected number of experts should be engaged for periods from one to three years for the carrying out of the several investigations and field experiences proposed. Experienced epidemiologists were to be invited to undertake the plague and cholera research as well as malariologists and public health officers devoted to their own specific field of expertise. Rajchman estimated a supplementary budget of $50,000 and enquired whether such a project would commit the Rockefeller IHD either as scope, duration or budget.

In addition the organization of the quarantine services in most Chinese ports was also assisted by the experts of the Singapore Bureau. Its personnel assisted as well in the organization and implementation of the campaign against cholera initiated in Shanghai and surrounding districts in accordance with a mission sent by the Health Organization of the League.

Annual reports for 1932 say that the Bureau had to deal with 188 infected ships, thirty affected by cholera, fort-four by smallpox and one by plague. While the weekly wireless information contained information concerning the measures taken by particular ports to protect themselves against infection, complete information on quarantine measures could not be supplied by this means and therefore full details were reserved for the weekly fasciculus, a bulletin published by the Singapore Bureau, containing information on the epidemiologic situation of Far Eastern countries, with records about the movement of passengers, quarantine measures taken, ports infected by plague and cholera or smallpox during the preceding twelve months.[109] By these means, the health administrations of 163 Far Eastern ports received updated information about the health conditions of the countries in the Region.

In 1932, the Government of the Union of South Africa requested the League to convene a conference on health problems associated to maritime navigation paying special attention to plague, smallpox and rural hygiene. The Director of the Singapore Bureau acted as General-Secretary of the Conference held in December 1932 in Cape Town. Through all this wide field of action, the Singapore Bureau achieved an established position in the field of international health work. Had it not been for the world economic depression, it was planned that the Bureau would be in 1934 maintained entirely by the Governments involved and by the League of Nations budget. This was the main argument: should the RF support cease at the end of 1934, the work of the Bureau would still be carried on but at a greatly reduced level. The RF did not neglect this important, transcendental and urgent demand.

The Global Centre of Documentation in Public Health

Previous pages show to what extent the availability of updated sanitary information was an essential issue for international health. As a result of the bilateral negotiations, in addition to the previously mentioned programs, a proposal for cooperation between the RF and the League of Nations in the establishment of a Centre for the Collection of Public Health Documentation was presented in May 1927 to gather documentation on public health activities all over the world: administrative reports, legal enactments, minutes of conferences and any other documents, manuscripts and publications.[110] Such a centre would have two principal functions: on the one hand the collection of important materials and, on the other, the spread and circulation of the information collected making it accessible to health authorities and public health experts. Information was conceived as an essential tool for the design of public health strategies. The materials to be collected, classified and analyzed would consist of documents, minutes of meetings, memoranda, printed and unprinted annual reports, the texts, decrees and regulations relating to public health in all branches and dealing with all possible countries: administrative reports, legal enactments, minutes of conferences and any other related publication. The 25 May 1927 minutes of the RF meeting session stated:

> A proposal for cooperation with the League of Nations in the establishment of a center for the collection of public health documentation was presented, as follows:
>
> 1 The proposal to establish a center for the collection of public health documentation is the outgrowth of the many inquiries originating within and without the Health Section of the League of Nations for information on the progress of particular phases of public health work in various countries. The Health Committee is expected also to advise the Assembly and the Council of the League in regard to international public health questions. Should a center of public health documentation be established, it would be possible to supply at relatively short notice detailed information on technical public health subjects for the use of the League itself or for such governments as desire it. It is believed that this service, if properly developed, would greatly increase the usefulness of the Health Section.
>
> 2 Such a center would have two principal functions: a. The collection of important material; b. The dissemination of information. The material to be collected, classified and analysed would consist of documents, minutes of meetings, memoranda, printed and unprinted annual reports, the texts, decrees and regulations relating to public health in all branches and dealing with all countries.[111]

Alfred Grotjahn, Professor of Social Hygiene at the University of Berlin, considered as one of the main founders of *social medicine,* was requested by the Health Organization to act as technical advisor of the new planned Centre for Public Health Documentation. He immediately expressed his acceptance to spend six weeks twice a year at the Geneva headquarters in order to advise the establishment and put into operation the new centre. Thereafter he spent the necessary time at Geneva and, on the basis of his experience, prepared a project, which was submitted to the Medical Director Ludwik Rajchman.

The first work on the organization of the Centre was started by a technical officer under the direction of a senior medical officer and helped by two assistants. The initial budget was $7,617.50 for the establishment, including salaries for a director, two clerks, a travel and technical advisor, purchase of documents and any other initial needs. In 1927 the RF contributed $6,937.50 for the Centre of Public Health Documentation during this year.

In March 1928 it was agreed to combine pledges for the International Epidemiological Intelligence Service and for the establishment of the centre of public health documentation conceived as complementary elements of a similar strategy involving the use of information on public health:

1928:	$60,335
1929:	$48,995
1930:	$44,155
1931:	$39,315
1932:	$34,475
1933:	$29,635
1934:	$22,400

Table 3.7: **Grant by the Rockefeller Foundation for the Support of a Centre of Public Health Documentation at the League of Nations, Geneva. Source: Rockefeller Archive Centre, NY.**

From 1930 to 1934, the RF contributed the huge amount of $700,000 and $2 million more to fund an ambitious library and a centre of documentation in public health at the League of Nations headquarters in Geneva. Nevertheless, the project was never fully implemented.

The HO was notified of the approval of this grant by a letter from the RF dated 16 June 1927. An initial sum of 6.937,50 SF was initially appropriated for 1927, and subsequently the grant was consolidated with other grants according to the following resolution of the RF Executive Committee:

That the pledges of February 10th and May 25th 1927, to the Health Section of the League of Nations for the Service of Epidemiological Intelligence and Public Health Statistics and the establishment of a Centre of Public Health Documentation be, and they are hereby consolidated in the amounts shown in the following schedule:

1928: 60,335 SF	1932: 34,475 SF
1929: 48,995	1933: 29,635
1930: 44,155	1934: 22,400
1931: 39,315[112]	

The Centre for Public Health Documentation would supply detailed information on technical public health subjects for the use of the League itself and for health administrations of the national governments. The material collected would consist of documents, minutes of meetings, memoranda, printed and manuscript reports and technical surveys, national and international legislation and any sort of sanitary regulations. The spread of the information collected would include the supply of information to the Health Committee and the Health Section and respond to enquiries from health administrations and periodical statements on the progress of various branches of health work printed by the Health Organization.

The first duties consisted of collecting and classifying all information then available and to supplement it where necessary according to the plan established by Alfred Grotjahn. There was a large amount of documentation in the Section consisting of detailed reports on the work done and working of the public health services in some twenty countries. All that documentation was supplemented by the information received from technical correspondents in thirty countries on the progress of public health work in those countries for the purpose of its inclusion in the *International Health Yearbook* and by the information collected by the various commissions of the Health Committee, as well as by reports prepared by members of the interchange program and fellows on their subjects of study.[113]

There was also a very considerable amount of information collected in the Library of the League of Nations, and it soon became evident that the Library was the place to house the Centre for Public Health Documentation. A Committee was set up in the Health Section to study the location of the Centre and, as result of the agreement reached, the whole documentation belonging to the Centre was transferred to the Library, where an assistant Librarian was in care of it.

In 1932 the work had progressed far enough to warrant taking a second step, namely to answer enquiries received from health authorities of the countries, public health officers, medical institutions and other experts or responsible persons. Therefore, a letter was sent in May 1932 to all health administrations and to the medical press of most of the countries, drawing their attention to the facilities existing in the Health Organization of the League of Nations for the supply of information regarding public health methods, strategies, technical reports, statistics and other technical papers regarding international health as well as sanitary conditions in various countries. Notice was also given that comparative information could be supplied about epidemiological records and statistics, as well as about national and international health regulations. In principle the enquiries attended were limited to those made by health administrations and the chiefs of national institutes and scientific research centres. Petitioners were asked to indicate the purpose for which the information was required.[114]

Since its creation onwards the Centre assisted a large number of requests mostly from health authorities of France, Bulgaria, Czechoslovakia, Switzerland, Russia, USA, Germany, Belgium, Spain and Argentina. The type of information required regarded the most relevant public health concerns: sanitary facilities, public health campaigns, nutritional problems especially among children, disinfection techniques, health insurance arrangements, lead poisoning, epidemiological records and health statistics, protection against dangers from X Rays, hospital architecture, water supplies, standards of vaccines, public health education, pasteurization of milk, tuberculosis, medical practice regulations and many others which constituted issues of sanitary concern at the time.[115]

After a first period of collecting documents and spreading the information requested, the necessity of amplifying the amount of information kept by the Centre and establishing new criteria of classification became evident. Better facilities were proposed for 1935, when the new Library rooms would permit a better settlement of the collection storage, the classification of a much larger number of documents and an easier access to a wide public. The value and usefulness of the Centre was soon well established and the only future difficulty was then an eventual reduction of the staff, which would make it impossible for any one member to devote enough time to the Centre and a hard management of the information collected, something that would not represent a serious problem except in the case that the Rockefeller Foundation finally would withdraw when the agreement ended on 31 December 1934. That was a blow to the expansion and improved continuation of the Centre.

Standardization of Biological Products and Food Rationing

In a broader sense, the term *standardization* applies to the development and implementation of concepts, procedures and laboratory practices to achieve and maintain the required levels of compatibility in operational and technical fields to prepare a substance for use and exchange.[116] Standardization was initiated in the context of less stable 'biologicals' like vaccines and sera and soon was extended to chemical drugs, being an essential starting point for the expansion of experimental biology. This generalization of the procedures implied as well the idea of a biological evaluation. The Paul Ehrlich Institute in Frankfurt became an international model for a quality control agency aiming to establish international standards and methods of evaluation.[117]

More and more, standards became the cornerstone of industrialization procedures. The increasing development of a health industry required standards for medicine production (vitamins, nutrients, etc.), but also to settle the borders between health and disease when analyzing body fluids and components, minerals, hormones, counting cells and tissue components and settling conventional relations between normality and health.[118] Something similar is to be said of the establishment of standards regarding children's development, nomenclature of causes of death, patterns to define the state and level of epidemics and many other aspects of health and disease that could be measured according to comparable results and applied to an international level. Laboratory medicine was grounded upon biological standards and, in the development of this path, the League of Nations played a meaningful role: it convened review commissions to boost negotiations and agreements, and special conferences and programs for the standardization of biological products.[119] The standardization program was among the most relevant of the League during the interwar years. Indeed, quality standards are an integral part of modern medical culture in the post-industrial world, and *Wertbestimmung*, evaluation procedures, constituted a recent quality control regime.[120]

The standardization of the efficacy of a given therapy or vaccine also served to circulate knowledge between medical researchers, clinicians, industrial producers and health administrators. The need to evaluate the quality of medicines of biological origin thus triggered the development of a specific procedure for testing their efficacy.[121]

Similarly to the Ehrlich Institute in Frankfurt a culture of quantification and standardization was soon introduced likewise at the Pasteur Institute, imposed by Émile Roux (1853–1933) and his co-workers as part of an approach to cope with the consequences of infectious diseases. Pasteur's approach to vaccination was limited by a time in which microbiology was still under construction and the shift to the development of immunological techniques had not yet started. The political conflicts dividing Europe into two main blocks did not really affect the collaboration between national research institutes of one side and the other and, after a first period of serious criticism and anti-German attitude in France, a new sociological environment appeared: Émile Roux and Émile Behring were friends and, both together with Iliá Metchnikoff, esteemed Robert Koch's scientific works. In this case, scientific research affinities were stronger than political and military confrontations.

After a first period of research on diphtheria antitoxins in most European institutes, the German standardization procedures were adopted and at the turn to the twentieth century, a more rational statistical analysis of the results obtained on therapeutic agents applied on humans was generally adopted. It was not merely the adoption of German standards of serum production against diphtheria from the Koch-Behring laboratories that was adopted by Roux-Duclaux as a simple transplantation of techniques; indeed, a reciprocal transfer of knowledge was taking place.[122]

The importance of standardization for public health, for a real international health and for the development of a global health industry, attracted the interest of the several agents. Regarding the Health Organization of the League of Nations; it is important to note that its medical director, the Polish Ludwik Rajchman, was a bacteriologist, and the president of the Health Commission, Thorvald Madsen, was the director of the *Statens Serum Institut* in Copenhagen and also developed the role of president of the Standardization Commission created by the League. Madsen had excellent contacts with serologists from both sides in Germany and on the allied side. Those details show the importance attributed to control and development of standardization by the leaders of the health sections of the League.

In December 1921, the Health Organization of the League held a Conference in London on the standardization of sera and serological tests, as the starting point of a general inquiry undertaken conjointly with the *Office International d'Hygiène Publique*.[123] Participants designed the Copenhagen's Institute as future caretaker laboratory replacing Frankfurt as central laboratory for sera and standards. Witherto the various systems of measuring and testing the strength of anti-toxins had been evolved independently of one another within different nations and even by different groups and institutes of research of the same nationality, thus causing much confusion and many difficulties for public health policies.[124] The creation of a uniform system of units of measurement was thus evidently a necessary piece of international medical cooperation that only an international organization endowed with enough legitimacy such as the League of Nations Health Organization could boost and coordinate.

The Conference was chaired by Madsen, who analyzed the problems involved in establishing common standards for diphtheria, tetanus, dysentery, anti-meningococcus and pneumococcus serum, and for the serum diagnosis of syphilis.[125] The meeting arranged a scheme for the international cooperation in carrying out the preliminary scientific investigations.[126] The Health and Serological Institutes of Austria, Belgium, France, Germany, Great Britain, Italy, Japan, Poland, Switzerland and the United States took part in the London Conference, and Dr Tarassevich, of the Russian Soviet Health Department, was prevented from attending due to bad travel communications. The Conference elaborated a program of enquiry and research, to be carried out by the different national laboratories, and then centralized in the Copenhagen Institute, acting as a clearing house for all the work. Results had to be examined and conclusions adopted at a fresh conference to be held at the Pasteur Institute in Paris. The big institutions of the most influential countries controlled the international process.

In certain remedies, biological products and sera, the doses could not be measured simply in relation to weight, owing to possible variations in the chemical composition and therapeutic potency. To ensure correct use of remedies, the RF and the LN promoted carrying out experiments on laboratory animals to agree on the *standard unit* of each remedy, that is to say the quantity, which produces a given effect upon an animal of a given species.[127] Due to the lack of international agreements, standards of drugs, pharmaceutical remedies, vaccines and serum differed widely in different countries, and this diversity caused scientific debates and trouble to medical practitioners and sanitary authorities when they had to deal with products from foreign origins. 'A doctor, for example, who is accustomed to administer 1.000 German units of a certain preparation to obtain a given clinical effect will only obtain negligible results with 1.000 American units, as the American units are one-third the size; this may involve serious risks for the patient'.[128] Therefore, the establishment of common standards for serums was preliminary to the most important task of exercising practical scientific control over the biological products in the market of international trade. The IHD appreciated the service rendered by the Laboratory of Hygiene in Washington in keeping under inspection vaccines and serums that were sent to the market and considered that something similar had to be done on an international scale. Therefore, the RF gave support to the standardization initiatives of the Health organization.

The growing tendency towards mass production and industrialization of the production of hormones, vitamins, drugs, vaccines among other pharmaceuticals, made the Rockefeller Foundation and the Health Organization of the League of Nations attach the greatest importance to the definition of international standard units for vaccines, sera and some other medical preparations.

Initial conferences held in 1921 and 1922 drew up a plan of work based on the constitution of a Permanent Standards Commission as the responsible board for the direction of research and international negotiations.[129] The method of work adopted could be summarized as follows: Once the project of standardization of a particular serum or medical product had been decided upon, the Commission usually started up by preparing a detailed scheme of research, which was entrusted to a series of prominent laboratories in different countries. The results were communicated to the Serum Institute at Copenhagen, which, in that case, acted as the central laboratory of the Health Organization of the League. When the experts of the Standards Commission determined that the results obtained were sufficiently clear to lead to definite conclusions, then a conference was appointed to summon the research experts in a space of negotiation at which any differences of opinion were easily discussed. In the exceptional case of difficulties remaining or lack of agreement among experts after this first meeting, the Commission drew up a new program of supplementary research, and therefore a second conference was appointed at which unanimous agreement was invariably reached.

Once a standard unit had been fixed and a method of comparison determined, one of the large public laboratories such as the State Serum Institute in Copenhagen, the Pasteur Institute in France, the National Research Institute in London, the Laboratory of Hygiene in Washington or the Institute of Experimental Therapy in Frankfort, was made responsible for the preservation of the standard on behalf of the Health Organization of the League of Nations. The power and predominance of those prominent institutes were absolute in the decision making process. This laboratory provided for the distribution of *standard units* to the various scientific laboratories, be they public or private, so that they could grade their products according to this *standard unit* which, thereafter the governments were requested to adopt officially in their pharmacopoeia, as a means of interchange and international agreement. This process opened the door also to international production of biological products and pharmaceuticals and to global trade.

In the matter of sera, during the first decade of functioning of the standards commission in the early 1920s, research was focused with a view to the standardization of anti-diphtheria serum and diphtheria antitoxin, the most efficient remedies at the time for the cure and prevention of this extended disease. Other researches focused on anti-dysentery and anti-tetanus sera, cerebral-spinal meningitis, scarlet fever sera and tuberculin vaccine.

The Health Organization had settled standard units for insulin, digitalis, pituitary extract and rye ergot, extract of male fern and oil of chenopodium, as well as arseno-benzenes and derivatives, used for the treatment of syphilis. Serological diagnosis of syphilis was also standardized through a test made of the blood serum of the patient, as a laboratory complement of the clinical examination. Border and Wassermann had developed a technique for syphilis serodiagnosis. Two conferences for laboratory experts were held in 1923 and 1928 to discuss sero-reactions, and a series of conclusive experiments were carried out and presented by sixteen specialists on almost one thousand tests.[130]

An international institute for the standardization processes of biological products under the League of Nations was built and settled in London, composed by members of the Permanent Standard Commission of the League ('permanent quarters for Standardization Commission'). Until then, the Copenhagen and the London laboratories acted as central laboratories for the League biological standardization work.[131]

The decision was taken immediately during the first meeting of the LNHO in 1921, when it was agreed working on standardization of sera and serological tests for syphilis. Madsen and Rajchman worked with determination towards international cooperation on sera standardization coordinated by the League. As a first step, Rajchman boosted an international conference of the expert serologists, which was held at the Pasteur Institute (1922). By late 1922 over thirty reports on standardization had been issued by the League. When the League's Standards list was reported in September 1935, the Permanent Commission on Biological Standardization had adopted International Standards for sera and vaccine products, glandular products, vitamins and therapeutic substances.

With the aid of the Rockefeller Foundation, the League of Nations boosted a wide, ambitious program for the standardization of biological products. The rhetoric claimed that technical committees were expected to behave as expert independent of national interests, 'free of all values except those of science'. Serologists were already an international community of like-minded experts that owed their own tradition and maintained a close collaboration, despite the international and political conflicts, and the immediate market interests.

Standardization of sera was urgent and biological standards were a sensitive matter. Since national institutes produced and distributed pharmaceutical standards, serological standardization required an international negotiation. Even before the Great War, Paul Ehrlich devised a solution combining several components, which required standardization methods: the preparation containing the active substance, the units expressing the measure of active substances, and the method of assessment. Although the Ehrlich Institute in Frankfurt assumed this task initially, its international influence became impossible for the political context during the Great War and in the meantime new units and tests for diphtheria and tetanus came into use and a confusing situation expanded. Conscious of the huge dimension and the importance of the problem, in 1921, the League coped with the problem. In June 1928 a Laboratory Conference on Sero-diagnosis of Syphilis gave meaningful agreements and in 1932, the Standardization Committee took up vitamins responding to demands of nutrition research.[132]

As time went by the importance of negotiations on sera standards declined due to the consolidation of international agreements, but the interests for standards for vitamins, hormones and pharmaceuticals increased. The pressure of the industry was a main factor. Collective security and control of hazards was always the rhetoric argument. The Inter-Governmental Conference on Standardization held in 1935 invited the national representatives to enter themselves into a system of government-approved National Centres under the two central laboratories in Copenhagen and Hampstead, to be responsible for receiving and passing on the standards to acceptable users. The arrangements were hurried into force when World War II broke out in 1939, although no treaty had been actually drafted and the war operated a change of direction representing a return to the government-oriented attempts to create a sort of standardized international system based on health regulations, as previously favoured by the Paris *Office International d'Hygiène Publique* and previously the International Sanitary Conferences during the second half of the nineteenth century.[133]

Between 1922 and 1935 the Standards Commission established international regulatory standards for eleven therapeutic sera, one bacterial extract, four vitamins, three sex hormones, five gland preparations and five other therapeutic agents. The target was to agree on standards and international units for important therapeutic substances requiring biological assay so that all large national laboratories follow the Commission's recommendations and applied its instructions in their national territories. In 1935 thirty-one countries had officially recognized and adopted the units and standards advocated by the Health Organization: nineteen countries in Europe, seven in America, one in Africa and three in Asia and Australia, preserving the principle of free distribution.[134] The work done into this direction during the interwar years was the first step leading to industrialization of biological products and to the establishment of regulations through national and internationals agencies for the validity of standards and patents.

The definition of dietary standards was an important milestone for the evolution of nutritional standards, for rationing policies and for the definition of the clinical forms of nutritional deficiencies and malnutrition, but the complexity of factors intervening in organic nutrition gave way to methodological controversies. A general agreement had not been reached either on the boundaries and clinical signs of *malnutrition* or on the methods to identify it in individuals under scrutiny. Paediatricians needed standards to determine children's normal development, and school medical officers requested simple working methods that could be applied to large groups of school children to spot those suffering from weakness, retarded development and chronic under-nutrition. Three different methods of assessing the *nutritional status* of the population were proposed. One was the comparison of certain bodily measures to a standard; another one was the assessment of the global state of health and development based on clinical screening; and the last one was a more refined clinical test to detect physiological problems and early deficiency diseases including laboratory analysis.

Although the height of a child depends to some extent on heredity aspects, long time faulty feeding could influence it. Comparing weight to standards was considered to be in general of little value, but the weight gain rate and the height-weight ratio were often used in assessing the nutritional status. *Indices of nutrition* established relationships between height, weight and other bodily measurements, although, concerning children, some experts preferred a simple comparison between the individual's weight and the average height for an age. A complete study would require laboratory techniques, not easily available in primary care checking and expensive to run on large groups. Simple *clinical methods* included careful examination of external features, a series of body measurements and the general examination of organs and systems.

The human organism needs to be supplied daily with a certain quantity of food energy that could be evaluated in terms of calories and therefore a considerable amount of research on calorie requirements was available in 1930s.[135] However a step forward was needed in the determination of dietary standards. Physiologists in previous decades had generally devoted their attention to *minimum dietary requirements*, also the usual standpoint of Governments when called upon to fix the rations to feed large numbers of soldiers and civilians in wartime, or to assist the unemployed and their families during periods of economic depression. But the idea of a *standard for an optimum diet* was developed during the 1930s, considering it as the one providing for the full development of the organism and for resistance to disease. Scurvy, rickets, beriberi or pellagra were considered clinical forms associated with nutritional deficiencies since the late 1920s and research on *standards for adequate nutrition* was essential to avoid deficiencies and to guide future dietary policies.

The Health Committee of the League aimed to reach an agreement among specialists on how the state of nutrition could be determined by means of a standard clinical examination. A Conference that convened to discuss this purpose in Berlin in December 1932 discussed two main issues: on the one hand the composition of diet and, on the other, methods for clinical examination. The second was regarded as the most reliable although it had to be applied to a sufficiently large number of people from various social groups. In the search of a definition of the borders of malnutrition, H. Laugier, expert of the Technical Commission of Nutrition of the League, proposed in 1936 a comparison between the weight at the moment of checking and the previous weight constituted. The amount of subcutaneous adipose tissue was also to be ascertained, but always taking into account that some obese individuals do not lose weight even if they eat very little and, conversely, there are thin people who do not put on weight notwithstanding a copious food intake.

The Technical Commission on Nutrition of the League approved in its third session (November 1937) a *General Report on the Physiological Bases of Nutrition* (1938) containing ten important topics regarding the nutrition of children and dietary standards. This report was strongly influential. It was communicated to learned societies, scientific institutions and national health authorities with a view to securing co-operation in the aforesaid studies.[136]

What constitutes a balanced diet? Answering this question means specifying the human requirements of calories, fat, proteins, vitamins and minerals and establishing the right proportions in which the various nutritional factors had to be combined. The nutritive value of food was to be the basis for dietary standards, which were the starting point for further practical action. They allowed assessment of the value of the diet of individuals, age and social groups, making it possible to draw up dietary schedules for those communities like armies, inmates at institutions, hospital patients, schoolchildren and prisoners. They were also used as the basis of large-scale wartime rationing schemes and as a starting point for future agricultural policies.

Human calorie requirements were investigated by calorimetric methods. The basal metabolic rate of an adult average European citizen was considered to range from 65 to 75 calories per hour, the energy exchange being lower during sleep and considerably higher during physical activities. As a result of laboratory research an average individual during an average day was found to need about 3,000 calories per day. This figure was widely used in practical interventions, put forward as a standard by the Advisory Committee on Nutrition of the British Ministry of Health and accepted by the most influential specialists. Energy requirements varied enormously according to the type of work performed, from about 6,000 or 7,000 calories in the case of a lumberman to 2,200 for a sedentary worker. The energy requirements of children and women were considered to be lower than those of an adult man. Both statistical and calorimetric data were registered for both sexes and age groups as the basis of *scales of family coefficients,* which calculated the needs of children and women in terms of an average man, the latter being taken as the standard unit. Such scales allowed the establishment of a *consumption unit* as a means to calculate the requirements of the entire group.

The agenda of the *Conference of Experts for the Standardisation of Certain Methods used in Dietary Studies* convened in Rome in September 1932, searching for an international agreement on a scale of *family consumption units.*[137]

The Expert Committee on Nutrition produced the following scale (1932):

Age	Male	Coefficient Both sexes	Female
0–2			0.2
2–3			0.3
4–5			0.4
6–7			0.5
8–9			0.6
10–11			0.7
12–13			0.8
14–59	1.0		0.8
Over 60		0.8	
		1.0 = 3.000 calories	

Table 3.8: **Calorie Coefficient by Age and Sex proposed by the Expert Committee on Nutrition of the League of Nations (1932). Source: League of Nations Archives.**

This international proposal was widely employed to make results easily comparable and to compare dietary habits and calorie intake in different countries. The Rome Conference also suggested that researchers engaged in dietary enquiries should, if possible, provide information not only with regard to the intake of calories, protein, carbohydrate and fat, but also about the intake of animal and vegetable proteins. Carl von Voit, German physiologist, professor at Munich and considered to be one of the founders of modern dietetics, made an initial proposal in his book *Food and the Principles of Dietetics* (London, 1927). He calculated that a man weighing about 70 kg and doing moderate work needs daily 3,055 calories, 118 gr. protein, 58 gr. fat and 500 gr. carbohydrates. Other standards proposed by physiologists, such as Atwater, Rubner and Hutchinson, did not differ significantly from the numbers proposed by Voit.[138]

The Mixed Technical Commission on nutrition of the League, International Labour Office and International Institute of Agriculture convened in London in November 1935 an issued a 'Report on the Physiological Basis of Nutrition' (1936). Edward Mellanby presided over the Technical Commission; E. Burnet and W. R. Aykroyd carried out a series of enquiries in different countries (United Kingdom, France, USA, Denmark, Sweden, Norway and the USSR) and R. Cathcart, an expert on quantitative methods, chaired the sessions. The main scientific aim was to reach a formula for an optimum human diet standard. According to the *London Report* (1936) a dietary standard had to take into account energy requirements, the proportion of protective foods and mineral and vitamin requirements. Foodstuffs were classified into two main groups: *protective* foods and *supplementary energy-yielding* foods. A *calorific method* was introduced to calculate individual needs according to tables based on *energetic quotients* so that calorie requirements could be assessed to ensure the healthy development of the human organism.

The standard for an optimum protein intake was under discussion during the 1930s. Some advocated a high intake while others restricted consumption. Contradictory clinical evidence about the effects of high protein diets on the kidneys contributed to the debate. Some experiments showed that diets containing 30 per cent protein produced signs of kidney damage in rabbits and humans, but those results had been criticized alleging that experimental diets were incomplete regarding dietary components other than protein. On the contrary, rats seemed to be in perfect health in other experiments after one year on a diet containing 70 per cent protein. General agreement arose on the fact that societies with a high protein intake have a better organic development than those with lower, but no inference could be drawn as to the optimum protein consumption.

In support of a low intake, many population groups consuming less than 70 grams of protein per day in rural areas of Europe were described as healthy, although others stated that little was known about vital statistics, resistance to disease or their physical potentialities with a richer protein diet. Some experiments claimed that health and nitrogenous balance could be maintained on a diet of cereals, potatoes, margarine and fruit containing only 32 grams of absorbable protein. One gram of protein per kilo of body-weight or about 70 grams for an average man was accepted but other specialists proposed a *protein standard* a bit higher of 100 grams. The Advisory Committee on Nutrition of the British Ministry of Health suggested 37 grams as a suitable daily allowance of 'first class' or animal protein for an average man, which would represent about 5 per cent of total calories on a diet yielding 3,000 calories per day. However some experts argued that there was no need to include proteins of animal origin in the human diet. It could be useful to include such proteins when the staple food covering energy expenditure was very poor in proteins and if these were low quality. The prejudice in favour of meat and luxurious dietary habits constantly increased the consumption of meat, something physiologically and economically inconvenient.

No knowledge had emerged in the interwar years as to the optimum proportions of carbohydrates and fats, although it was accepted that they were interchangeable within wide limits. Carbohydrates were acknowledged not only to provide energy, but also to facilitate the breakdown of protein and assist the metabolism of fat.

The following standards were proposed in 1935:

	Protein	Fat (grams)	Carbohydrate	Calories
Voit	118	56	500	3,055
Rubner	127	52	509	3,092
Atwater	125	125	450	3,520
Advisory Committee (British Ministry)	100	100	400	3,000
Playfair	119	51	531	3,140
Tyszka	80–100	60–80	500	3,000

Table 3.9: **Standard Dietaries put forward by experts in physiology of nutrition. Source: E. Burnet and W.R. Ayckroyd, 'Nutrition and Public Health', *League of Nations Quarterly Bulletin of the Health Organization*, 4:2 (1935), pp. 323–474.**

Moreover no diet could be considered adequate by the expert nutritionists unless it contains all mineral elements present in human tissues taking part in metabolic actions, which need to be replaced by nutrition. An International Vitamin Conference was held in London in June 1931 under the auspices of the Permanent Commission on Biological Standardization of the League's Health Organization. A further report was published in 1934 on international standard units for vitamins A, B1, C and D, and another report was issued in 1937 by the Technical Commission on Nutrition of the League summarizing available knowledge on mineral, vitamin, protein, fat and nutritional requirements during the first year of life including a table on the nutritive value of food.

In August 1938 the Technical Commission on Nutrition met in Geneva. The experts convened under the chairmanship of Mellanby, Secretary-General of the Medical Research Council, London. The meeting dealt with the nutritive value of cereals according to the degree of milling, the influence of climate on food requirements, and the extent to which diets in common use fell below the standards recommended in the *Report on the Physiological Bases of Nutrition* (1936). As a result of the economic crash in 1929 and the deep depression a great deal of the population saw their income wane and some energy requirements calculations were published: 2,500 calories was considered to be the daily average requirement of an unemployed man.

Family Unemployed	**Calorie Requirements**		**Calorie**	**% Reduction**	
	Strenuous	Moderate	Unemployed	Strenuous	Moderate
Single man	4,000	2,800	2,500	39	11
Man & Wife	6,400	5,200	4,900	23	6
Man with two dependants (wife and child of 10)	8,500	7,300	7,000	18	4
Man with three dependants (wife + 2 children 9 & 5)	9,400	8,200	7,900	13	3

Table 3.10: ***Report on the Physiological Bases of Nutrition*** **(Geneva: League of Nations, 1936).**

Subsequent to the international situation during the interwar years, war and post-war times and during the economy depression, problems related to diet arose and community feeding became essential. An increasing section of the population claimed food relief and a considerable part received meals in residential institutions, armies, hospitals, sanatoria, prisons, asylums, schools, canteens and other similar institutions. Several systems for the provision of cheap meals extended previous experiences. In France the *soups populaires* and the *fourneaux économiques* were enlarged; in Germany, *Caritas Association* lent its kitchens to volunteers in 1932 in cities such as Cologne to provide meals for thousands of people. In Britain the provision of meals through central city kitchens, traditionally used for school-meals and nursing mothers, was extended and in some cities like Birmingham the *Citizens' Society* founded a number of canteens in occupational centres run by the unemployed. Something similar happened in Spain with school canteens and social kitchens for the poor.

In accordance with dietary standards food rationing policies were introduced in most European countries as an early measure even before scarcity had time to develop. Rationing systems were designed to secure an equitable distribution of the available supplies of essential foods to all the population. In addition, food rationing sought to supplement and reinforce measures of price control and production planning, something necessary for managing the economy of war. Without effective coordination between the various phases of the social and economic policy, particularly between the availability of supplies, an organized system of distribution and price control, food rationing could not work smoothly. In this case, thanks to the experience gained with the Great War and the Spanish Civil War. On the basis of the latest developments in the experimental science of nutrition, European governments were remarkably successful in managing their rationing policies, a central aspect of the political economy in war time.

Two main models of rationing were standardized and applied during World War Two, conceived by the experts according to their suitability to the economic situation of the country involved. One was the *German-type*, also called *Continental,* and the other one the *Anglo-American-type*.[139] The German system represented an improvement of rationing schemes as they were applied during the Great War. It was adopted all over the European continent with some particular modifications depending on local characteristics, availability of foodstuff, agricultural production etc. This rationing system was conceived according to a stringent supply situation. Food imports to Europe accounted for 10 per cent of the supplies before the conflict, but they were entirely cut off, whilst the production of domestic crops contracted to approximately 80 per cent of the normal standards by the end of the war.[140] Therefore, the problem in continental Europe was the capacity to satisfy the nutritional requirements of the whole population, the total food consumption, according to nutritional requirements and an efficient distribution of foodstuffs to the whole population. The solution of this challenge was sought by introducing a reduction in livestock, transferring to human consumption a greater part of the crops released from animal feeding. This policy resulted in a lower animal-vegetal ratio in the diet, with a higher proportion of vegetable calories being consumed.[141]

However, in considering the nutritive value of the diet, it was extremely important not to reduce excessively the proportion of animal proteins and calories, provided that some of them – as in the case of milk for children – were deemed to be essential for health, to maintain organic defenses, to avoid undernourishment and to secure the adequate organic development of infants and children. Under the German-Continental rationing system any important foodstuffs were particularly rationed in amounts per person, per day, per week or per month. In some cases a family scheme was also implemented. Rationing was the system applied by nutritionists to guarantee both the minimum quantity and the essential quality of diets. Indeed, the logic of markets in times of scarcity tended to trigger an increase of prices and produce maladjustments and social exclusion. As a counterbalance strategy, rationing tried to avoid foodstuffs becoming too expensive and diets too low in daily calorie intake.

A plurality of factors had to be considered in order to adjust rationing to the needs of the population groups. Physiological needs for food varied in a significant degree according to sex, age and occupation, and therefore, rationing tried to be made differential to minimize inequalities. To do so, the rationing schemes used to divide consumers into several categories, each one receiving rations in proportion to previously calculated physiological needs. But the number of categories was limited for practical and administrative reasons, and as a matter of fact the system did not fully eradicate inequalities, at least in terms of calorie intake.[142]

Moreover experts were aware of the negative attitudes of the population towards rationing inasmuch as it represented a break in previous traditional dietary habits and limitation to the free market of foodstuffs. Therefore, to be successfully accepted, rationing required a highly efficient administrative apparatus and also the support of the public opinion. When those fundamentals were missing – and this applies especially to the procurement of food from farmers – an increasing proportion of the total food supplies were shifted to the more attractive and lucrative black markets, a main threat for the proper functioning of the system.

From a pure medical and physiological perspective, the efficiency of rationing was directly proportional to the amount of calories that the rations afforded. Qualitative or cultural elements – i.e. the prestige or bad reputation of certain foodstuffs associated to consumption by upper or lower social groups – were not taken into consideration. In accordance to official international reports,[143] on the whole, rationing proved efficient throughout the war in Germany, Czechoslovakia, Denmark, Sweden and Switzerland, and also in the Netherlands for most of the time, but it was less successful in countries such as Belgium, France and Norway. In southern and eastern European countries, rationing collapsed altogether at the end of the war. Official records about the real consumption were hard to collect at the end of the war, since under conditions of extreme scarcity, as was the case with Greece in 1943, the black market supplies entered the scene and were not easily evaluable.[144]

The situation was quite different in the United Kingdom, where rationing schemes were never sealed off during the war. Although access to overseas supplies was seriously threatened, rationing was chiefly introduced in order to husband the scarce shipping space and foreign trade. The domestic output was directed towards the production of bulky or perishable foods, such as wheat, vegetables and milk, whilst food imports were primarily directed towards providing for concentrated animal products. Throughout World War Two no absolute limitation of the supply of total calories took place in Britain. The consumption of bread and most vegetables remained without any limitation, operating as a sort of *budget regulator* permitting consumers to purchase as many calories and foodstuffs as they required if they could afford them. On the other hand, rationing was designed not to guarantee a minimum balanced diet, but to distribute scarce foodstuffs such as animal products, sugar and fats equally.[145] It was devised so as to meet the average needs for all the main nutrients, and considered that there was no need for a differential calorie rationing, basic rations being based on an equal *per caput* allocation.

Some specific population groups required quality foodstuffs. This was taken into account by the implementation of special distribution schemes, separate from the general rationing system. In this respect, reference must be made to special rations of milk and protective foods for children, for nursing and pregnant women and specific arrangements for community feeding initiatives and for canteens for industrial workers. Additional, non-essential rations were also supplied by the so-called *point-rationing* system. This method ensured a fairly wide consumer's choice between different commodities. Indeed, the Anglo-American system remained more flexible than the German-Continental system throughout the war and, therefore, it was better adjusted to individual choices and traditional family habits. On the whole, rationing was limited to animal foodstuffs, mainly to prevent the uneconomic expansion of animal farming products, while providing for a sufficient amount of export, lend-lease and military needs.[146]

In critical times of hunger and political crisis, research on dietary standards was boosted by national governments becoming the background for rationing schemes and public health policies. During the 1930s the LN developed a fundamental role in the coordination of international research groups and expert commissions. Consequently the traditional meaning of diet as something simply associated with cultural traditions was transformed according to a more scientific and political perspective. Traditional dietaries became carefully scrutinized according to physiological patterns, and dietary standards were the instrument as well as the tool for measuring dietary needs and community nutritional policies. This phenomenon is closely related to the huge expansion of food industry and to the starting point of the so called *nutritional transition.*

4 INTERNATIONAL HEALTH AND THE END OF THE LEAGUE OF NATIONS: GAUTIER'S EVALUATION

The German expansion during the early 1940s deeply affected all of the programs of the League of Nations and its sections dispersed: the Economic and Financial Section as well as the Transit Section moved to Princeton, the Treasury and Refugees Departments were settled in London, the Drug Traffic Department in Washington and the International Labour Office in Montreal. However the Health Section remained at the *Palais des Nations* in Geneva. In addition, due to exceptional circumstances, hardly any country paid their contributions to the budget, considering the League of Nations as a diplomatic agency was obsolete and defeated by the extraordinary conditions of the wartime. Those days the budget consisted almost entirely of British Commonwealth payments and some reserve funds. As a matter of fact, by 1941, the budget was only a third of what it had been during the years prior to the war.[1]

During the first years of the conflict, the League lost the majority of its principal leaders and experts:

> As of June 1940, the Section consisted only of a handful of left-over people: Raymond Gautier, Swiss public health expert and Yves Biraud, French expert for epidemiology, and a small clerical staff. The continuation of the League of Nations Health Organisation for the following four years rested on their shoulders. They could not expect a lot of support from the Health Committee members. Thorvald Madsen, the Health Committee president for nineteen years, wrote two postcards in German from occupied Copenhagen saying that he was fine and that his institute continued producing sera, but that it was impossible for him to come to Geneva. There would be no more news from him until the end of the war. Meanwhile, his Belgian colleague in the Committee, René Sand, was deported to Germany. Committee President Parisot, was captured but released in October 1940. He returned to France, but did not contact the Section until April 1941. Inexorably, Gautier's and Biraud's efforts became a struggle for institutional survival.[2]

By 1943 negotiations started in order to set up of a future International Health Agency (IHA) linked to the new international organizations that were under negotiation among the big powers to operate after the end of the war. Gautier received a request to write an outline for the future International Health Agency and he contributed his personal views out of any League commitment.

Gautier answered the request and wrote an outline in which he defended that the future IHA should be unique and autonomous, overcoming the evident limitations of the dependence of the Health Organization from the League. A Swiss expert in public health after being director of the University Institute of Hygiene and Bacteriology at Geneva, Gautier joined the League of Nations in 1924, where he initially was concerned with biological standardization. Between 1926 and 1930 he acted as director of the Far East Bureau in Singapore and when he returned to Geneva he devoted his efforts again to the standardization program. In 1939 he became acting director of the Health Section and from 1942 until the end of the war he was entrusted with missions to London and Washington for the purpose of organizing public health in the liberated territories of Europe. When the World Health Organization Interim Commission became established in 1946, Gautier became first counsellor, a few months later he was appointed Director of the Geneva Office and in 1948 he assumed the role of Assistant Director-General of the permanent Organization until his retirement in 1950. Gautier was a prominent figure in the design of the World Health Organization based on his decades of experience in the League Health Organization.

During wartime it was assumed that the *Office International d'Hygiène Publique* in Paris was controlled by Germany and it would not be worthwhile to recover it after the war since 'its utility and efficiency were debatable'.[3] Already in the moment of writing his outline in 1943 Gautier considered unlikely the survival of the League of Nations after the War, although he saw indications that use could be made of its technical organizations as a base on which to build the new model for an international health agency. He stressed the experience achieved in international health, the amount of documents and reports sampled, expertise gained in Geneva and consequently that simple logic indicated that the wide network of collaboration achieved over decades should not be dismantled and wasted. In many senses, the new organization could not be so different because most of the work was considered positive and the international dimension of health problems remained.[4]

Gautier proposed selecting from among the Paris and Geneva health policies those which had proved useful and welding them into a logical and workable scheme. Nevertheless, the future IHA should have higher aims, greater power and heavier responsibilities than the Health Organization of the League. 'For health is more than the absence of illness: the word "health" implies something positive, namely, physical, mental and moral fitness. This is the goal to be reached; but it lies beyond the possibilities of curative and preventive medicine'.[5]

As a matter of fact, for historical reasons the organization of the League was not the result of a well-planned decision, but the consequence of the difficult circumstances in interwar years. The scheme based on an advisory board

(*Office International*), a leading organism (Health Committee) and an executive agency (Health Section) was logical at the time, although the reasons to adopt such a model did not exist in 1943 and, subsequently, the new IHA was conceived avoiding adverse factors, taking advantage of the previous experience and widening the fields of activity.

Gautier recognized the necessity of keeping and improving a global service of epidemiological intelligence and expressed a much positive opinion of the pioneer work done in Geneva and Singapore. The International Epidemiology Intelligence Service was to become the model of a world centre for the tabulation of epidemiological records and vital statistics. Regarding the circulation of epidemiological information, Gautier advocated to simplify procedures and minimize the interference of diplomatic agencies avoiding any sort of confidentiality to epidemiological information following the example of the Far East Bureau. Difficulties or irregularity in collecting the required information were supposed to disappear as all the health administrations were under the authority of the IHA, making the notification of plague, cholera, smallpox, typhus and yellow fever compulsory, and reporting all diseases will therefore no longer be dependent on a state having ratified the Sanitary Convention. Gautier recognized that introducing compulsory notification of minor epidemic diseases was too ambitious and unrealistic at that stage at a global scale, but he insisted on that direction and considered that if IHA should keep close watch on the world's health, it must be able to follow the extent and outbreaks of influenza, eruptive fevers, diphtheria, meningitis, poliomyelitis, enteric fevers and dysentery. In the early 1940s information on the prevalence of those diseases was limited only in certain countries and large municipalities endowed with a solid health administration, and therefore it should be the aim of the IHA to improve the situation and generalize the reporting of those diseases, as well as other important social diseases such as tuberculosis, cancer and sexually transmitted diseases. The report did not mention explicitly tropical diseases, probably because during wartimes the focus was mainly put on the reconstruction of European countries.

Gautier advocated for the continuity of epidemiological publications in order to furnish at a glance a view of the world's state of health, something which implied a close collaboration with the International Institute of Statistics at The Hague regarding the standardization of lists of causes of death and its global acceptance. Whilst Geneva would remain the world centre for epidemiological intelligence, branches in each continent were set up with a view to acting as collecting and broadcasting agencies, reopening the Singapore Bureau for Asia and Australia. Although the Alexandria Bureau had ceased functioning in 1941, Gautier thought that there was no need to resuscitate it since the central site in Geneva could assume the epidemiological control of the Near East and North Africa regions. For the rest of the African Continent, it was urgent to establish a regional bureau, and the Pan-American Sanitary Bureau in Washington, the recognized centre of information for the Americas, continued its work. This scheme, based on the existence of a world centre of epidemiological intelligence in Geneva, was embodied in the new International Sanitary Convention, which would have to be drafted as soon as possible to substitute the old one signed in Paris in 1926.

In addition to public health problems such as the collection and treatment of epidemiological information and negotiations on quarantine regulations, many other issues required international approach, but Gautier insisted on the fact that public health, and particularly international health, in order to be effective after such a convulsive period should be, as much as possible, free from direct political interference. Usually the approach to health problems required specialized knowledge and this could best be achieved by the establishment of committees of experts, as done by the League during its twenty years of existence. Complex subjects such as biological standardization, the fight against malaria or nutritional policies against malnutrition and rationing systems had been successfully tackled due to the scientific authority of experts. Following previous experience, Gautier suggested international conferences as another positive formula for the negotiation of scientific matters.

Notwithstanding, Gautier expressed critical opinions regarding the deficiencies of international health in previous time. He thought that in the past the choice of subjects to be approached internationally not always had been sufficiently discussed and the best options chosen. He believed that out of the numerous subjects worked out internationally so far hardly any had been dealt with exhaustively, even those which had accumulated important amounts of experience.[6] The whole field of epidemic and contagious diseases had been explored both from the curative and preventive perspectives with a satisfactory degree of success, but other important social diseases had been neglected or very little taken into consideration. As a matter of fact, Gautier mentioned cancer as an important issue lacking of an international comprehensive plan of action, likewise the rules governing prevention of tuberculosis, which had to be updated, and a scheme for the treatment of syphilis was to be convened after the progress made in the serological diagnosis of the disease. Gautier claimed for an authoritative statement regarding the principles along which an anti-venereal campaign should be run, including the problem of prostitution in its sanitary and moral dimensions.[7]

Malaria and rabies were also mentioned in Gautier's report as requiring international attention. The value of the work done by the Malaria Commission of the League derived mainly from the fact that the problem was faced on the field deserving knowledge of the local conditions and this scheme could also be advantageous for other diseases. Another issue, research on rabies had been mainly focused on the standardization of vaccines after the Rabies Conference held in 1926 and Gautier claimed for a second conference to make new decisions.

There was a general opinion that the standardization of biological products had reached an increasing global importance and should be boosted in the future. Therefore the IHA should take over the program and national health administrations should be compelled to adopt the twenty-seven biological standards established so far. In 1935 an intergovernmental conference had summarized recommendations in this field, but they had not been applied on large scale yet. As we know, during the League of Nations activities, the Hampstead and Copenhagen Institutes had acted as principal centres for the preparation and distribution of biological standards. Nevertheless, Gautier proposed the creation of one world centre invested with the necessary administrative and scientific authority out of national involvement. An attempt was made in London by 1930 to concentrate this program and, after the war, London or the USA could be a good election, according to Gautier's opinion.[8]

The Health Organization had the initiative of a plan for the unification of requirements inserted in national pharmacopoeias as to the purity of the principal drugs. More than a hundred proposals had already been drafted as a basis for the shaping of an international pharmacopoeia and a successful conclusion was yet to be achieved. Following this initiative, Gautier proposed the suppression of the International Secretariat of Pharmacopoeias acting those days in Brussels under the Belgian Government and the integration in the new International Health Agency.[9]

Beyond the urgent relief policies for refugees during and after the war, living and health conditions in rural districts and migrations from and towards the cities were further important issues involving health policies. The Health Organization had promoted conferences on rural hygiene in Europe, Asia and Africa during the 1930s, a subject which had reached higher importance as a consequence of the disasters caused by the war and the impairment of living conditions and health standards. In a time when the 'return to the land' policy was advocated in many countries this program could not be left aside, especially considering the hard living conditions of peasants and the necessity to improve living standards in rural districts.

Certainly Gautier believed that similar considerations had to be applied to nutritional policies. Severe food restrictions were expected during the post-war years and the creation of an international food board to minimize malnutrition and famine was an evident necessity, although this initiative became soon frustrated due to the particular economic interests of the big international powers.[10] After relief, reconstruction was the next step and a proper nutrition and food availability was considered to be, more than any other social reform, the essential issue of social stability and growth. Before the creation of FAO, Gautier proposed a coordination of the IHA with the National Nutrition Institutes established in most countries to share information about large-scale consumption studies, dietary standards for the various climatic conditions to be formulated and the establishment of liaison with the economic, agricultural and transport world authorities. Once more, experts in nutrition should play a relevant role following the predominantly technical approach defended by the League leaders.[11]

The housing program to be drawn up as a consequence of the war disasters required going far beyond the repair of war damage, but also at the improvement of rural life. Urban planning, illumination, safe water supplies and other factors linked to local conditions and alien to public health were involved, but the implementation of sanitary standards was essential and IHA had an important role to play.

Once more, going to the experts, adequate instruction of public health specialists and officers was still considered to be an essential factor and that is why the Health Organization devoted so much attention to the instruction of experts, interchange programs, coordination of national public health schools, training of malariologists and other similar activities. From the perspective of 1945, the IHA should not be reluctant to follow the same path considering public health experts as cornerstone of the national systems and international action.

The usefulness of an international health agency was reinforced by the numerous requests for technical help received in the headquarters of the League in Geneva from health administrations during the two decades of work of the Health Organization. As Gautier stated:

> The following examples will show the diversity of the problem raised: reconstruction of the health services of China, Greece and Czechoslovakia; sanitary survey in Bolivia; control of syphilis in Bulgaria; anti-cholera campaign in Shanghai; control of malaria in Albania, Siam and Yugoslavia; anti-typhus action in Rumania; nutritional survey in Chile. Obviously, similar requests will be addressed to the IHA, which should be able at any moment to deal with them. Some will require expert advice only; others will necessitate surveys on the spot or even field work. The personnel required will need to have various qualifications according to the nature of the request, and the IHA should know to whom it can apply in case the demand exceeds the possibilities of its own staff. This requires permanent liaison with experts specialised in various subjects, as was done by the Health Organisation.[12]

Gautier thought that the future agency should even go a step forward and take the initiative of intervening when international solidarity required it without waiting for a government request as it happened after the Great War when the Epidemics Commission intervened in Poland. This was always a controversial issue.

Moreover for social stability in the new times, social security could not be conceived without a system of health insurance and medical care for all. Gautier was convinced that sooner or later this would come about and the IHA should pull the experience gained and serve as an advisory centre, although he recognized this was a delicate ground in each country for several reasons:

> On the one hand, health insurance has for years been the undisputed preserve of the International Labour Office. On the other hand, medical treatment for all raises the hotly debated question of State Medical Service versus private practice. The whole

> status of the medical profession may be at stake; for if medical care for all is to be realised, a complete preventive and curative service must be provided, and inability to pay should not determine people from benefiting by it. The IHA may not be asked to take sides in the controversy, but I cannot ignore it.[13]

The plurality of national options after the war and during the Cold War years regarding health care will show to what extent Gautier's assessment was right. Health education was another field of action, where there was still much to do. Gautier proposed that the IHA should assemble a film library and even take the initiative to produce films trying to introduce health education at schools and in youth movements, similar to what the Red Cross Societies have done in this direction. Ultimately, the IHA should serve as well as a world centre of information and a clearing house for the discussion of public health problems and this required a well-organized library, an efficient archive and a centre of documentation updating information, creating abstracts of essential contributions and doing a proactive policy of diffusion of information.

Although the establishment of an IHA was universally accepted, a crucial aspect was to be discussed and a solution adopted in order to avoid the proposals and decisions of the IHA remaining simple ideas and that they were actually put into effect. And this directly touched the authority in front of the political autonomy of the states. Even in such a crucial moment as it was at the end of the world war, it was doubtful that a Government could be urged, or even compelled to enforce sanitary measures for solidarity and international security. A general principle applied international agreements when interfering with national affairs and therefore no external imposition was accepted by the states. Public health experts endowed with an international perspective thought that orienting certain national health policies towards social progress would find strong resistance among certain powerful elites and Gautier was extremely clear on this issue:

> It is high time, however, that quarantine and even the fight against epidemic diseases should cease to be considered as the alpha and omega of the public health. Curative and preventive medicine, although they have certainly not exhausted their possibilities, cover one aspect of the problem only. Instead of specialising in the defensive, health policies should be constructive in the sense of bringing to the people something most of them have lacked so far. The possibility of integral health.[14]

In his thoughtful report Gautier showed his criticism on the results of some previous experiences. The Paris *Office d'Hygiene Publique,* having enjoyed solid political status and responsible government delegates, was, however, constraint by a political dependence and an academic and very restrictive approach to practical health problems, lacking of expert knowledge and showing desperate slowness in its responses.[15] On the contrary, the Health Organization of the League had many advantages in the manner how technical problems were dealt with, setting up expert commissions and the more technical the subject, the better the results obtained. Gautier mentioned the results achieved in three outstanding fields: standardization of biological products, malariology and nutrition. To be successful, political independence was a cornerstone to enable and carry out this work and international authority should be recognized beyond political options.

When he wrote his report, by 1943, there were some sixty independent States in the world, out of the colonial dependencies, and this political landscape was about to change very quickly. Compulsory affiliation with the IHA was assumed, but States were not to take an active interest in international health work in so far as they derive a practical advantage from it. Otherwise, Gautier considered that some powers would adopt a distant indifference more obstructive and destructive than showing an open and frank opposition.[16] In the search of a definition of health problems at a regional, local and global scale, providing the IHA with a regional decentralized structure would be more effective. Thus Europe, America, Australasia and Africa would each have their own health council and Gautier suggested Geneva, Singapore and Washington as administrative centres leaving open the choice for the most suitable option for Africa. Although the Continental Health Councils should enjoy a high degree of autonomy, their activities would need to be guided and coordinated by a central organism. This World Health Board (or whatever the name adopted, which was finally, as we know, World Health Organization), should therefore be so highly qualified as to be recognized as the supreme authority on health matters. Gautier conceived the WHB as a technical body of highly qualified experts and hygienists of international reputation and its democratic functioning was very important. Therefore, the question of allotting votes would require special attention:

> Should the same value be attributed to the vote of any one country, irrespective of its importance and degree of development? In other words, should the views of Paraguay carry the same weight as those expressed by Canada? Anomalous as this equality of rights may appear – and the League has had bitter experience of it –, I would be reluctant to suggest that a coefficient be attributed to each country, especially if it were to be proportionate to the size of the annual contribution paid, as was the case of the Paris Office. Anyhow, it is likely that a similar problem will arise in other branches of international activity, and it will be for the 'Over-All World Authority' to decide on a uniform policy.[17]

Gautier summarized his scheme for a future IHA in six principal points. His opinion and the importance of his report is easy recognizable in the foundational principles of the World Health Organization Acts, which stated:

1. There was a recognised need for an International Health Agency.
2. The Health Organisation of the League should serve as a nucleus for the International Health Agency.
3. The International Health Agency should be unique and safeguarded from political interference, getting integrated into the scheme of a new world organisation.

4 The International Health Agency should aim at securing positive health for everyone, as a prerequisite to freedom from want and social security.
5 The administrative structure of the International Health Agency should be based on the regional principle.
6 The activities of the Continental Health Councils should be directed and coordinated by a World Health Board, which would act as technical adviser to the Over-All World Authority.[18]

Gautier signed his report in London in 15 March 1943. In such a critical moment, the document expressed his experience as leading authority of the Health Organization of the League and provided the core ideas, which served to conceive the architectural foundation of the World Health Organization a few years later on the ashes of the League of Nations Health Section.

5 SOME GENERAL CONCLUSIONS

When the Health Organization of the League of Nations was established in 1921 general doubt prevailed as to what extent it would be possible to justify its existence, the usefulness and capacity of influence of international health work and whether it would be forthcoming from the public health services of all nations in any part of the world. Financial support was essential for its continuity and not easy to obtain, but at this initial stage the political support was the most decisive factor. After the first campaigns to fight epidemics in Poland and Russia, and later on, when the first results were achieved, particularly as regards the standardization of biological products, International Epidemiology Intelligence Services and the Interchange of Public Health Officers, the Health Committee was encouraged to take a lead increasing the extent of the programs. The support of the Rockefeller Foundation was then an essential factor, to the extent of a *condition sine qua non* for the big programs guiding the activities of the Health Organization during the interwar period.

After two years' work the health authorities of many governments came to appreciate the usefulness of international health work and after 1926, national governments began to apply to the League for advisory recommendations and technical help, for the creation of special commissions or for the investigation of public health problems of particular significance. The strategy followed by the medical director and most active figure of the HO policies, Ludwik Rajchman, consisted of obtaining the collaboration of the best-qualified specialists, sometimes not easy to recruit for the League because they were engaged in research institutions or national health policies. Good medical training, university distinctions, administrative experience in public health, international background and knowledge of languages, as well as certain diplomatic skills were essential for the establishment of an active framework of public health experts coordinated by the RF and the League. The RF was fully aware in 1926 of the importance of technical competence and involving excellent officers from various nationalities, including British, American, French and German, who were also members of the Health Section.

The agreement and the financial support of the RF was not only essential in order to allow for the stabilization of the LNHO activities, but also to preserve intact the technical team of public health workers responsible for the executive activities of international public health work. The work of the Health Section was considered by the RF leaders as being a systematic effort to use public health activities for political stabilization to gain closer understanding between the various governments of the world. The strategy was clear, the LNHO was not to get engaged in promoting directly laboratory research or scientific discoveries, but its scope as a public health international organization was the practical application of the results of research advances as it is in consonance with the program of national health administrations.

George Strode, the head of the International Health Division of the Rockefeller Foundation in Europe during a part of the interwar years, reported in 1936 to the New York central office a general overview of the public health work done by the League of Nations Health Organization during the previous fifteen years of collaboration. He was absolutely proud and positive about the work done:

> Some day the history of public health in Europe, since the Great War, will be written. When it is, it seems likely that the schools and institutes of hygiene are destined to bulk large therein, both in significance and in importance. There are twenty-five countries in Europe, exclusive of the British Isles and Russia, and fourteen of them are equipped with national schools of institutes of hygiene. It is interesting to note that in ten of the fourteen the International Health Division has cooperated in the creation of these institutions. The ten countries are Bulgaria, Czechoslovakia, Denmark, Hungary, Italy, Norway, Poland, Rumania, Turkey and Yugoslavia.
>
> Reliable investigators who have inspected and assessed the schools and institutes declare them to be the most valuable contribution that has been made to present-day public health in Europe.[1]

Obviously, the quality and the efficiency of both the schools of public health and the national institutes of hygiene in the instruction of public health experts and in national health policies were closely linked to the high qualification of the staff. If they were to be classified as to their excellence and value, they would in no ways follow size or modernity of equipment and facilities but would show a positive correlation to the competence and enlightenment of the directing personalities. The human factor was essential. This simple fact was, of course, clearly appreciated by the IHD officers when the collaborative programmes were discussed and, as a consequence, aid was not mainly limited to the material aspects, but concerned itself equally with the high quality of the personnel involved. The program of fellowships and travel grants was awarded to a large number of the experts who subsequently held responsible positions in the technical and administrative branches of the national health administration.

Initially there was a certain degree of uniformity in the training programs and practical experience of the public health experts, since they studied in more or less similar schools and got their practical experience through contact with the same technologies and field activities. The interchange of programs and experiences for national schools of public health was very fruitful in order to exchange experiences and find similarities in the organization and administration of public health institutions and in the concepts and procedures applied by their directing personnel.

In all but one of the fourteen countries participating in the program – the exception was Romania – the schools of public health and institutes of hygiene were conceived and brought to fruition by the health administration and not by university schools of medicine, though it would have been logical for them to have developed from university chairs of hygiene. The explanation was easy to understand: for centuries the universities had trained physicians for a curative oriented medicine, but they did not have the tradition in training for preventive medicine. Although chairs of hygiene and public health were created in most European universities since mid-nineteenth century, only British Universities met the challenge of creating schools of hygiene. Romania fell behind Great Britain but in the rest public health grew under the dependence of the public administration.

The political importance of public health and social medicine during the interwar years made the question arise as to whether this system of specialized training in public health was the best and should persist in the future. The loss of political importance of preventive medicine after World War Two, as a consequence of the emergence of the sanitary industry and the foundation of national health care systems based on a more curative perspective, minimized the importance of this question giving rise to a powerful hospital medicine. The hospital became the locus of an endless technological innovation in medical care. Experts cconsidered that if medical care was to become a legally acknowledged right of every citizen, in the same sense as education, medicine would become increasingly preventive and the training of medical practitioners and public health officers would be drawn close together, and the schools of hygiene more closely associated with schools of medicine. Although the events would show in the future that this foresight was not successful, in the meantime, preventive medicine was assumed and supported by government authorities, which recognized the value of specialization and of competence in public health. They thought that the better and the stronger these schools came to be, the more easily they would fit into the university environment.

The Rockefeller Foundation played a dominant role in creating and boosting such training institutions. Its success and its failures have usually been foreshowed by local circumstances. Hungary was considered a splendid example of the success of the International Health Division policy as it was recognized in internal reports of the American Foundation. In his last annual report for 1935, the director of the National Institute of Hygiene of Budapest recognized that the establishment of the institution was made possible only with the help of the grants of the Rockefeller Foundation. The importance of the institute was best proven by its capacity to cope with the economic depression, keeping activities and the commitment of the Public Health Administration and assuring the constant development of the

Institute. Nevertheless the involvement of the Rockefeller IHD in public health reached other activities than simply schools of public health and institutes of hygiene. The IHD funded grants for the organization of health departments and boosted practical actions to cope with such diseases as malaria, scarlet fever, schistosomiasis, influenza and yellow fever in different countries and regions.

Moreover, its scope became increasingly globalized. During 1936 the mandate of the Paris Office was extended to include all of Africa, as well as Europe and the Near East. The expansion in those regions was compensated in part by the end of a series of active programs in a number of European countries. During the period of 1930–5 projects were developed and implemented in nineteen European countries, whereas there were but eleven of these in which work, aside from fellowships, was carried on in 1937. The new regions of Africa and the Near East added three countries to the active project list: Cyprus, Egypt and Uganda.

In 1936, the Rockefeller authorities expressed a certain degree of satisfaction upon withdrawal from a given country, as it was an indication that the original objectives had been attained and that conditions were favourable to prosecution of the work by local authorities. This was the Rockefeller experience with programs in England, Ireland, Norway, Denmark, Holland and Yugoslavia.[2] The situation was also assessed as very positive in Republican Spain, but during the course of 1936 the RF was forced to withdraw from Spain due to the war circumstances. 'Whether an opportunity will subsequently be presented to continue aid and to bring the several projects to fruition in that country, time alone can tell. For the present, we consider them terminated and fresh negotiations will be called for prior to renewing IHD interest and responsibility'.[3]

There were two countries added to the IHD list in 1936 in which there had not previously had a program supported by the Rockefeller Foundation. The first, Belgium, was surveyed and contacts were started to be included in the RF fellowship program. In due course projects were to be developed looking towards an improvement in its public health organization and administration. The other country, Uganda, offered the IHD an opportunity to develop, cooperatively with it a yellow fever research institute. The proposal was accepted and by the end of 1936 the organization of the research institute was nearing completion.

> These two countries, five days apart by air and three weeks by rail and sea, illustrate the two dominant features of the IHD program today. On the one hand, a program orientated towards the improvement and modernisation of state and local health services and, on the other, the field investigation of a disease of world importance, in the hope of bringing it under control through greater knowledge of its natural history and the discovery of means whereby it may be successfully combatted.[4]

The Rockefeller International Health Division enlarged during the second half of the 1930s its field of action. Ten new projects were initiated. Four of them could be classified as studies or investigations related to certain specific diseases including malaria in Cyprus, influenza in Hungary, yellow fever in Uganda and a subsoil irrigation project to fight schistosomiasis in Egypt. With the exception of the prompt schistosomiasis project in Egypt, the other programs were likely to be continued over a period of years. In addition three more projects were classified as surveys including the previously mentioned survey about the Belgium's public health organization, a survey on nursery training facilities in London and a survey regarding Hungary's public health facilities. Except the last mentioned, these surveys were of short duration and terminated during 1937. The remaining three of the ten new projects were the Bucharest School of Nursing, the Local Health Service in Tirana and Developmental Aid to the Ankara School of Public Health, which involved aid to experimental work in sanitation, minor sanitary engineering and eventually epidemiological studies as well. The Rockefeller International Health Division planned special studies and investigations along with surveys as the dominant new activities, without an abandonment of the previous interest in state and local health departments of public health education. At that time the IHD RF functioned as a sort of philanthropic advisory services for international public health requests of the different countries around the world.

When the Spanish Civil War started, the Rockefeller authorities made an account of the Spanish situation and they concluded that most of Rockefeller projects in Spain were terminated. Only a program of research on vaccines developed at the National Institute of Hygiene, closely linked with research projects at the Rockefeller Institute in New York, was maintained. As a matter of fact, the working programs in most of the European countries were completed in 1936. These comprised of seven projects under the heading 'state and local health work'; five classified under 'public health education', which included aid to the *Bulletin of Hygiene*, developmental aid to Schools of Hygiene in Warsaw and Zagreb, aid to the building and equipment of the Prague School of Nursing and the survey of nurse training facilities in London, as well as five investigations and programs of intervention on specific diseases such as diphtheria, malaria, smallpox and tuberculosis.

Collaboration conducted over two decades between the International Health Division of the Rockefeller Foundation and the Health Organization of the League of Nations was an essential instrument for the internationalization of public health, the establishment of permanent networks of international diplomacy around health and the settlement of a large network of public health experts, fully communicated through conferences, institutional cooperation and political programs. The technical approach to public health problems and the spirit of dialogue and negotiation are probably two of the greatest contributions to the expansion of international health policies according to the pattern of social medicine based mainly in epidemiology and health statistics, standardization of methods and values and experimental research. That was the core of the collaboration between the Rockefeller Foundation and the League of Nations. Their collaboration was an outstanding chapter in the history of public health and a milestone in the process transforming health as a powerful element in international diplomacy.

APPENDIX 1: INTERNATIONAL SANITARY CONFERENCES, COMMISSIONS AND BOARDS, PREVIOUS TO THE LEAGUE OF NATIONS (1920)

INTERNATIONAL SANITARY CONFERENCES, COMMISSIONS AND BOARDS PREVIOUS TO THE ESTABLISHMENT OF THE LEAGUE OF NATIONS **(1920)**[1]

1835: International Sanitary Board, Tunisia (1839)
1838: International Sanitary Board, Constantinople
1840: International Sanitary Board, Tangier
1843: Health, Medicine and Quarantine Board, Alexandria
1851–2. International Sanitary Conference, Paris
1852: 1st International Congress Hygiene and Demography
1856: European Commission for Danau (sanitary agreements).
Congrès Internationational de Bienfaissance, Correction et Philantropie
1859: International Sanitary Conference, París (1959)
1863–4: Red Cross International Centre, Geneva
Red Cross National Societies
1865 y 1866: International Sanitary Conference, Constantinople
1866: General Sanitary Intendance, Alexandria
1867: International Conference on Tuberculosis
1st International Medical Congress
(Exposition Universelle, Paris)
1874: International Sanitary Conference, Vienna
1888: International Conference on Tuberculosis, Paris
1889: International Congress on Medical Health Care
1893: International Sanitary Conference, Dresden
1894: International Conference on Tuberculosis, Paris
1897: International Sanitary Conference, Venice
1898: International Conference on Tuberculosis, Paris
1899: International Conference on Tuberculosis, Berlin
1899: International Office to fight women and children traffic
1900: International Conference on Tuberculosis, Naples

1902: Central International Office to coordinate fight against Tuberculosis
1902: Pan-American Health Office, Washington
1903 y 1911: International Sanitary Conference, París
1907: Office International d'Higiène Publique, Pars
1920: International Sanitary Conference, London
League of Nations Health Committee

APPENDIX 2: HEALTH SCHEME OF THE LEAGUE OF NATIONS FOR THE ESTABLISHMENT OF A PERMANENT INTERNATIONAL HEALTH SECTION

Health Scheme of the League of Nations for the establishment of a permanent International Health Section[1]

Organization

It is hereby proposed to establish a permanent International Health Section as part of the Organization of the League, to deal with those Public Health questions, which for the sake of all countries require International consideration and standardized action.

Permanent Organization

This shall consist of:
An International Health General Committee
An Executive Committee
An International Health Office

The General Committee

The General Committee shall consist for the present of delegates appointed by the Governments represented on the Committee of the Office Internationale d'Hygiène Publique, and may therefore include representatives of Governments not as yet signatory to the Covenant of the League of Nations, but who have signed the Convention of Rome of 1907.

The General Committee shall appoint its own President, regulate its own procedure, and may at any time appoint sub-committees to consider any special question. Any delegate may at any time call in the assistance of technical advisors. The advisors shall not speak except at a request made by a delegate whom they accompany, and by a special authorization of the President of the Committee, and they may not vote.

A delegate however, who may for any particular reason be unable to attend, may by notice in writing addressed to the President appoint an adviser to act as his deputy, and his advisor while so acting shall be allowed to speak and vote.

The general Committee shall meet from time to time as occasion may require, not less than once in every year, and for the present at the Headquarters of the Office Internationale d'Hygiène Publique in Paris, unless otherwise decided by a vote of two thirds of the Committee.

The Official languages of the International Health Section shall be French and English.

The Executive Committee

The Executive Committee shall consist of not more than nine members of whom one shall be the President of the General Committee, one a representative of the League of Red Cross Societies and one a representative chosen by the Governing body of the Labour Conference.

The remainder shall be elected by the General Committee and should be persons having technical knowledge of the Public Health Service of their countries.

The Executive Committee shall elect its own Chairman and regulate its own procedure, but shall meet not less than four times a year, and may in addition at any time be called to deal with questions requiring urgent consideration. It shall be empowered to form sub-committees and to call in technical advisors on special points, but these advisors shall have no voting power.

Full reports of the proceedings of the Executive Committee and of all sub-committees shall be submitted to the General Committee.

The Chairman and Members of the Executive Committee shall hold their appointments for three years only, but shall be eligible for re-appointment or re-election.

The International Health Office at the Seat of the League of Nations

This shall consist of:
Be appointed by the Executive Committee, and as far as possible with due Staff

The *Medical Secretary* shall be appointed by the Executive Committee, and shall be responsible to this Committee for the efficient working of the International Health Office, and for any other duties as may be assigned to him by the Executive Committee. He shall have the right of direct access to the Secretary General of the League of Nations, and be empowered to have direct communication with all Government Health Offices.

He shall be entitled to attend all meetings of both Executive and General Committees, and shall be a member ex-officio of all Committees.

The *Staff* of the International Health Office at the seat of the League of Nations shall (on the recommendation of the Medical Secretary) be appointed by the Executive Committee, and as far as possible with due regard to the efficiency of the work of the Office, shall consist of persons of different nationalities.

The Headquarters of the International Health Office shall be at the seat of the League of Nations.

The *Office Internationale d'Hygiène Publique*

Subject to the approval of the Government signatory to the Rome Convention of 1907, the *Office Internationale d'Hygiène Publique,* shall IN VIEW OF THE PROPOSED CONSTITUTION OF THE GENERAL COMMITTEE, be merged in the new International Health Organization, under the direction of the League of Nations. Its existing establishment shall continue for the present in Paris.

Members of the General and Executive Committee, and of the Staff of the International Health Office shall have the right to use the Library of the *Office Internationale d'Hygiène Publique,* and its rooms in Paris shall be available for special meeting if required.

The Bureau of the *Office Internationale d'Hygiène Publique* shall undertake such new duties as may be assigned to it by the Executive Committee, in accordance with the resolution agreed to by the Committee of the *Office Internationale d'Hygiène Publique* at the meeting held in Paris on October 30th, 1919.

The Committee of the *Office Internationale d'Hygiène Publique* will agree to such alterations as may be found necessary in the *Statuts Organiques* of the Rome Convention of 1907 (especially article 15) and in the rules governing the internal administration of the Office, especially Article 8 of Part 1 of these rules, but no alteration shall be made in Part 2 with regard to the 'Caisse de Retraite et de Secours du Personnel'.

Expenses

The Expenses of all new Organization, Special Commission and Establishment Charges of the International Health Office of the League of Nations shall be paid from the Consolidated Funds of the League.

The Medical Secretary of the International Health Office shall prepare in advance a quarterly statement of all expenditure for his Executive Committee, whose responsibility it will be to recommend sanction for the proposed expenditure to the Secretary-General of the League of Nations.

The Medical Secretary shall be responsible to the Secretary-General of the League of Nations for the proper expenditure of all monies paid to him and shall submit to such audit as may be deemed desirable.

Until otherwise determined the expenses of the *Office Internationale d'Hygiène Publique* shall be paid as at present by contribution according to the appointment of the Rome Convention.

The League of Nations will concern itself with the collection of these contributions from the various members concerned. An annual estimate and statement of expenditure shall be drawn up by the Director of the *Office Internationale d'Hygiène Publique* in consultation with the Medical secretary of the International Health Office and his Executive Committee, and shall be forwarded to the Secretary-General of the League of Nations.

The *Office Internationale d'Hygiène Publique* shall from time to time submit to such auditing of expenditure as may be deemed desirable by the Secretary-General of the League of Nations.

Functions of the International health Office

These will be to deal with such matters as affect individual countries only in their relation to other countries.

These main functions may be summarized under the following headings:

To advise the League of Nations in matters affecting health.

To bring Administrative Health Authorities in different countries, into closer relationship with each other.

To organize means of more rapid interchange of information on matters where immediate precautions against disease may be required (e.g. epidemics) and to simplify methods for acting rapidly on such information where it affects more than (one) country.

To provide a ready organization for securing or revising necessary Internal agreements, for administrative action in matters of health, and more particularly for examining those subjects which it is proposed to bring before the executive and General Committee, with a view to the conclusion of International Conventions.

To be advisory to the International Labour Office on Health questions.

To confer with, and when requested to advise the League of Red Cross Societies and other authorized voluntary organisations.

Conventions

The Executive Committee shall be empowered to draw up any draft new Convention or revise existing ones.

These Conventions must, however, be submitted to the General Committee for consideration and approval, and a majority of two thirds of the votes of the General Committee will be required on the final vote for the adopting of the draft Convention.

In framing any Convention, the Committee may, in all cases, obtain the advice of Technical Trade experts when the matter is in any way likely to affect International Commerce. If it be decided that the draft Convention shall be adopted it shall be signed by the President of the General Committee and the Medical Secretary of the International Health Office, and then be deposited with the Secretary-General.

Each Member undertakes to bring the draft Convention before the authority, within those competence the matter lies, for the necessary action before one year has passed for formal ratification.

Any Convention so ratified shall be registered by the Secretary-General of the League of Nations, but shall only be binding upon the members who ratify it.

Each member of the General Committee agrees to make an annual report on the measures it has taken to give effect to the promises of the Convention to which it is a party.

These reports shall be circulated to all members of the General Committee, and shall, in addition, be given publicity in the Press, if necessary.

In the event of any member failing to carry out this undertaking the Executive Committee reserves to itself the right of putting in a report on the matter for consideration by the Council of the League of Nations, who will decide that action shall be taken.

The Government in question shall, however (if not already represented on the Executive Committee) be entitled to send a representative to take part in the proceedings of the Committee while the matter is under consideration.

Signed: R. Crowdy
H.Q. League of Nations
12 December, 1919
[RAC, RG 1.1., series 100, box 20, folder 165]

APPENDIX 3: AGREEMENT BETWEEN THE LEAGUE OF NATIONS HEALTH ORGANIZATION AND THE INTERNATIONAL HEALTH BOARD OF THE ROCKEFELLER FOUNDATION

ARTICLES OF THE AGREEMENT BETWEEN THE LEAGUE OF NATIONS HEALTH ORGANIZATION AND THE INTERNATIONAL HEALTH BOARD OF THE ROCKEFELLER FOUNDATION

September, 1922

1. This Agreement is made between the League of Nations, acting through its Secretary-General, on the one hand, and the Rockefeller Foundation, acting through the Executive Committee of the International Health Board, on the other hand, for the maintenance of an International Interchange of Public Health Personnel on an international scale.
2. The Health Organisation of the League of Nations will establish and maintain an International Interchange of Public health Personnel as a separate branch of its work, to begin operations on October 1st 1922, or as soon thereafter as possible, and to continue for not less than three years unless by mutual agreement between the League of Nations and the Rockefeller Foundation some other arrangement is made.
3. The work of the Interchange of Public Health Personnel shall be conducted along the following general lines:

To bring public health administrators in different countries into closer relationship with each other.
To make comparative examination of the organisation of the legislation regarding public health in different countries.

The endeavour to obtain the cooperation of the public health administrations for the purpose of agreeing upon a uniform standard of public health and uniform regulations.
It is necessary accordingly:

(1) To organise meetings of public health officials from various countries, and to make it possible for these officials to remain for a certain time attached to the health services of their countries, so that
- a They may have opportunities of exchanging views on health problems
- b They may have opportunities of acquainting themselves with the public health organisations of those countries, and with the manner in which the regulations are applied and with the duties of the health officials.

(2) To make grants towards the expenses of sending from time to time a small number of public health officials to study on the spot the public health organisations in other countries, and the manner in which the regulations are applied and the duties of the health officials.'
(3) Study of the simplest and most reliable methods of obtaining information regarding the incidence of disease and the progress of epidemics.
(4) Comparative study of public health statistics of different countries.
(5) Study of the world distribution of particular diseases.
(6) Comparative study of the incidence of particular diseases in different countries and their public health statistics, with a view to determining the nature and practical significance of observed difference between them.
(7) Study of the periodicity of epidemics and the factors, which cause or influence such periodicity.
(8) Organising, with the concurrence of the public health administrators of the countries affected, missions of enquiry regarding the development of epidemics ...
(9) The publication and distribution of special reports and periodical bulletins.
(10) A review of the public health of the principal countries of the world ...
(11) Organising a rapid interchange of information in regard to particular diseases in cases in which immediate action appears to be necessary.
(12) The employment at headquarters or elsewhere of experts provided with requisite assistance and technical equipment'.[1]

4. Annual reports of the administration of the Interchange of Public Health Personnel will be rendered to the Council and Assembly of the League of Nations, and copies of these reports will be forwarded regularly to the International health Board of the Rockefeller Foundation. Representatives of the Rockefeller Foundation will be kept closely and regularly informed of the activities of the interchange of public health personnel.

5. The Rockefeller Foundation agrees to pay an annual subvention to meet the expenses of the interchange of Public health Personnel, not to exceed 60.080 dollars a year for each of the three years 1922/23, 1923/24 and 1924/25.

6. The Rockefeller Foundation agrees to pay the annual subvention in quarterly instalment, beginning October 1st, 1922, directly to the Financial Director of the Secretariat of the League of Nations.

7. The Financial Director of the Secretariat of the League of Nations will administer the subvention paid by the Rockefeller Foundation as a separate Fund for the maintenance of the Interchange of Public Health personnel, to be known as the Interchange of Public Health personnel Fund, and will make disbursements from this Fund at the direction of the Secretary General of the League of Nations, after a budget has been approved by the Health Organisation of the League.

8. The special accounts of the Financial Director for the Interchange of Public Health personnel Fund will be audited as directed by the Council of the League of Nations.

9. Annual statement of account of the Interchange of Public Health personnel Fund will be rendered to the Council and Assembly of the League of Nations, and copies of these statements will be forwarded regularly to the International Health Board of the Rockefeller Foundation.

10. The present articles of Agreement may be modified bu the mutual consent of the Council of the League of Nations and the Rockefeller Foundation.

11. These Articles of Agreement have been approved by the Council of the LoN and will become effective on their approval by the International Health Board of the Rockefeller Foundation.

WORKS CITED

Primary Sources

Sources

League of Nations Archives, Palais des Nations, Geneva.

Annual Report of the Health Organization, 1925, C.H. 442 (A.17.1926.III).

Annual Report of the Health Organization, 1926, C.H. 529 (A. 9.1927.III).

Annual Report of the Health Organization, 1927, C.H. 682 (A. 10.1928.III).

Annual Report of the Health Organization, 1928, C.H. 783 (A. 8.1929.III).

Annual Report of the Health Organization, 1929, C.H. 863 (A. 7.1931.III).

Annual Report of the Health Organization, 1930, A. 7.1931.III.

Audit of the Accounts for 1930 of the Grants of the Rockefeller Foundation Towards the Budget of the Health Organization. (Communicated to the Assembly, the Council and the Members of the League), A.3(a).1938.X.

Audit of the Accounts for 1937 of the Grants of the Rockefeller Foundation towards the Budget of the Health Organization. (Distributed to the Members of the League, the Assembly and the Council), A.3(b).1931.X.

Epidemiological Intelligence Conference (Geneva, 1927), C.H. 663.

European Health Conference (Warsaw, 1922), C.I.E. 1–C.I.E. 50.; C.177.M.96.1922.

Health Committee. Report by Dr. Carozzi on the work of the Health Service of the International Labour Office. Geneva, League of Nations, 1923, C.H.86.

Health Committee. Eighth session held at Geneva from Wednesday, October 13th, to Tuesday, October 19th, 1926. Geneva, November, 27th, 1926, C, 610.M. 238. 1926. III.

Health Committee. Eleventh session held at Geneva from October 28th, to November 3rd, 1927. Geneva, December 15th, 1927, C.579.M.205.1927.III.

Interchange Grants financed by the Rockefeller Foundation, 1928, C.H. 701.

Interchange of Public Health Personnel, 1925, C.H./E.P.S./71.(1).

International Conference on the Biological Standardisation of Certain Remedies (second) (Geneva, 1925), C.H./C.P.S./P.V.

International Conference on the Standardisation of Sera and Serological Tests (London, 1921), League of Nations Archives, C.533.M.378.1921.III.

International Conference on the Standardisation of Sera and Serological Tests (second) (Paris, 1922), League of Nations Archives, C.H./S.S. 1 – C.H./S.S. 32.

International Health Conference (London, 1920), Minutes, 10/51/1–20/51/8.

Invitation from George G. Strode to J. Avenol, to the Regional Presentation of the International Health Division of the Rockefeller Foundation, July 1, 1938, 8A/2493/546.

League of Nations, Information Section, *The Health Organization of the League of Nations* (Geneva, 1931).

League of Nations Starts, The: An Outline by Its Organisers (London: MacMillan and Co. Ltd, 1920), on https://archive.org/stream/leagueofnationss015671mbp/leagueofnationss015671mbp_djvu.txt [accessed 27 May 2013].

Letter from the Health Section of the League of Nations to L. Rachjman, 19th November, 1924, 12B/54915.

Letter from S. M. Gunn to N. White, November 27 1925, 12B/56015/91838.

Letter from F. Read to Selskar M. Gunn, 12 November 1926, 12B/56915/21836.

Letter from Deputy Secretary-General to S. Gunn, March 12 1927, 12B/57957/21836.

Letter from Dr Dale to L. Rajchman, 28 November 1928, 8E/9865/9865.

Letter from G. K. Strode to L. Rajchman, June 5 1930, 8A/36608/M 716.

Letter from G. K. Strode to F. G. Boudreau, November 12 1931, 8A/36608.

Letter from L. Rajchman to G. K. Strode, 29 September 1932, 8A/36608/569.

Letter from L. Rajchman to G. K. Strode, 14 November 1932, 8A/36608/569.

Letter from G. K. Strode to L. Rajchman, December 13 1932, 8A/36608/569.

Letter from G. K. Strode to F. G. Boudreau, October 3,1933, 8A/546/X.

Letter from S. M. Gunn to J. Avenol December 28 1938, 8A/9493/546.

Letter from S. M. Gunn to R. Gautier, November 23 1939, 8A/2493/546.

Minute Sheet from the Treasurer of the Rockefeller Foundation, 8 February 1927, 12B/56915/21836.

Premier rapport de la commission de contrôle à l'Assemblée de 1936. Genève, Société des Nations, le 25 Mai 1936, A.5.1936 X.

Provisional arrangements made for the interchange of public health personnel during 1924. League of Nations Health organisation, C.H. 139 (C.H./E.P.S./31).

Provisional Health Committee. Provisional Statute of the Health organization. H.S.1–H.S.7.

Report by Dr. Carozzi on the work of the Health Service of the International Labour Office. Geneva, 11 May 1923, C.H.86.

Report of the Health Committee to the Permanent Committee ... ', A.22.1924.III.

Report to the Council on the Work of the Twenty-Fourth HC Session, February 1937, C.148.M.96.1937.III, pp. 11–12.

Report to the Council on the work of the twenty-Fifth session of the Health Committee (Geneva, 26 April – 1 May 1937). C.291.M.159.1937.III.

Resolution of the International Health Board Containing Pledge to Make Contributions to the League of Nations Service of Epidemiological Intelligence and Public Health Statistics, 11 February 1927.

Suggested draft letter from the secretary-general of the League of Nations to the International Health Board of the Rockefeller Foundation. League of Nations Official Journal, November 1922, 1256.

Technical Conference for Consideration of Certain Methods of Biological Standardisation (Edinburgh, 1923), League of Nations Archives, C.H./B. 1- C.H./B. 3.

Technical Laboratory Conference on the Serodiagnosis of Syphilis (Copenhagen, 1923), League of Nations Archives, C.5.M.1924.III.

Vérifications des comptes pour 1935 relatifs aux sommes reçues de la Fondation Rockefeller au titre de contribution au Budget de l'Organisation d'Hygiène. Genève, Société des Nations, 1936.

Work of the Health Committee during its fourth session, The (14–21 August 1922), C.594. M. 374. 1922. III.

Rockefeller Archive Centre (RAC)

Boxes and Folders

RG 1.1, series 100, box 20, folder 164 (Minutes 1922–34).

RG 1.1, series 100, box 20, folder 165 (1922).

RG 1.1, series 100, box 20, folder 166 (1923).

RG 1.1, series 100, box 20, folder 167 (1924).

RG 1.1, series 100, box 20, folder 168 (1924).

RG 1.1, series 100, box 20, folder 169 (1925).

RG 1.1, series 100, box 20, folder 170 (1926).

RG 1.1, series 100, box 20, folder 171 (1927).

RG 1.1, series 100, box 20, folder 172 (1928).

RG 1.1, series 100, box 21, folder 173 (June–December, 1928).

RG 1.1, series 100, box 21, folder 174 (1929).

RG 1.1, series 100, box 21, folder 175 (1930).

RG 1.1, series 100, box 21, folder 176 (1931–2).

RG 1.1, series 100, box 21, folder 177 (1933).

RG 1.1, series 100, box 21, folder 178 (1934).

RG 1.1, series 100, box 21, folder 179 (1935–6).

RG 1.1, series 100, box 21, folder 180 (1938).

RG 1.1, series 100, box 22, folder 181 (1938–41).

RG 1.1, series 100, box 22, folder 182 (1942–4).

RG 1.1, series 100, box 22, folder 183, League of Nations Health Section, Reports 1922–5.

RG 1.1, series 100, box 22, folder 184, League of Nations Health Section Reports 1926–34.

RG 1.1, series 100, box 22, folder 186, League of Nations History, 1946–8.

RG 1.1, series 100, box 22, folder 187, League of Nations History, 1949–54.

RG 5, series 1. Correspondence, subseries 2 Projects, box 273, folder 2899.

RG 5, series 1. Correspondence, subseries 2 Projects, box 273, folder 2902.

RG 5, series 1.2, box 273, folder 3466, Correspondence-Project.

RG 5, series 1.2, box 273, folder 3459, Correspondence-Project.

RG 6.1 (Field Office-Paris), series 1.1 (Prewar-Correspondence), box 37, folder 462 (League of Nations-Eastern Bureau).

RG 6.1, series 1.1, box 38, folder 471 (1930–8).

RG 6.1, series 1.1, box 38, folder 466 (1930).

RG 6.1, series 1.1, box 38, folder 468 IHD League of Nations-Permanent Standardization Commission (1934–8).

RG 6.1, series 1.1, box 38, folder 473.

RG 6.1, series 1.1, box 38, folder 477.

Documents

Correspondence, RAC, RG 5, series 1, subseries 2 Projects, box 273, folder 2899.

Correspondence, RAC, RG 5, serie 1, subseries 2 Projects, box 273, folder 2902.

Correspondence-Project, RAC, RG 5, series 1.2, box 273, folder 3466.

Correspondence-Project, RAC, RG 5, series 1.2, box 273, folder 3459.

Crowdy, R., *Health Scheme of the League of Nations (6th draft)* 12/12/1919, by Rachel Crowdy, Secretary-Gral of the League of Nations, RAC RG 1.1., series 100, box 20, folder 165.

'Dr Syssin's Summary of General Situation and Prospects for Working with League of Nations. Report of the Sanitary Epidemiologic Section of the Commissariat of Public Health Referring to Struggle with Cholera', RAC, RG 1.1, series 100, box 22, folder 183 (1922–5).

'Epidemiological Intelligence Service', RAC, RG 1.1, series 100, box 20, folder 165.

Gautier, R. Report on 'International Health of the Future', RAC, RG 1.1, series 100, box 22, folder 182 (1942–4).

'Grant for Training in Methods of Vital and Public Health Statistics', RG 1.1, series 100, box 21, folder 174 (1929).

'Grant for the Maintenance of a System of Interchange of Public Health Personnel on an International Scale', RAC, RG1.1. Series 100, Box 21, Folder 175, 1930.

'Grant by the Rockefeller Foundation for the Establishment and Upkeep of the Health Organisation's Eastern Bureau at Singapore', RAC, RG1.1. Series 100, Box 21, Folder 175 (1930).

'Grant by the Rockefeller Foundation for the Support of a Centre of Public Health Documentation', RAC, RG1.1. Series 100, Box 21, Folder 175 (1930).

Gunn, S. Memorandum by ... RAC, RG 1.1, series 100, box 20, folder 170 (1926).

IHD League of Nations-Permanent Standardization Commission (1934–8), RAC, RG 6.1, series 1.1, box 38, folder 468.

League of Nations-Eastern Bureau, Field Office-Paris , Prewar-Correspondence. RAC, RG 6.1, series 1.1, box 37, folder 462.

League of Nations Health Section, Reports 1922–5. RG 1.1, series 100, box 22, folder 183.

League of Nations Health Section Reports 1926–34. RG 1.1, series 100, box 22, folder 184.

League of Nations History, 1946–8. RG 1.1, series 100, box 22, folder 186.

League of Nations History, 1949–54. RG 1.1, series 100, box 22, folder 187.

Letter from E. Drummond to W. Rose, 2 September 1922, RAC, RG 1.1, series 100, box 20, folder 165.

Letter from G. Buchanan to T. Madsen, 27 July 1922. RAC, RG 1.1, series 100, box 20, folder 165.

Letter from L. Rajchman to W. Rose, 1922 RAC RG 1.1, series 100, box 20, folder 165.

Letter from S. Gunn to F. F. Russell, 12 October 1923, RAC, RG 1.1, series 100, box 20, folder 166.

Letter from S. Gunn to F. F. Russell, 14 February 1924, RAC, RG 1.1, series 100, box 20, folder 167.

Letter from F. F. Russell to S. Gunn, 13 March 1924, RAC, RG 1.1, series 100, box 20, folder 167.

Letter from F. F. Russell to S. Gunn, 15 April 1924, RAC, RG 1.1, series 100, box 20, folder 167.

Letter from F. F. Russell to S. Gunn, 11 October, 1924, RAC, RG 1.1, series 100, box 20, folder 168.

Letter of N. White to F. F. Russell, 20 November 1924, RAC, RG 1.1, series 100, box 20, folder 168.

Letter from Eichel to Russell, 30 May 1924, RAC, RG 1.1, series 100, box 20, folder 167.

Letter from F. M. Read answered to Eichel, 20 June 1924, RG 1.1, series 100, box 20, folder 167.

Letter from S. Gunn to L. Rajchman, 2 September 1924, RAC, RG 1.1, series 100, box 20, folder 168.

Letter from L. Rajchman to S. Gunn, 3 September 1924, RAC, RG 1.1, series 100, box 20, folder 168.

Letter from L. Rajchman to S. Gunn, 8 September 1924, RAC, RG 1.1, series 100, box 20, folder 168.

Letter from L. Rajchman to S. Gunn, 25 September 1924, RAC, RG 1.1, series 100, box 20, folder 168.

Letter from L. Rajchman to S. Gunn, 14 February 1925, RAC, RG 1.1, series 100, box 20, folder 169.

Letter from D. B. Wilson (Ministerio de Instrucción y Salubridad Públicas) to F. F. Russell, 15 June 1925, RAC, RG 1.1, series 100, box 20, folder 169.

Letter from S. Gunn to F. F. Russell, 28 August 1925, RAC RG 1.1, series 100, box 20, folder 169.

Letter from S. Gunn to F. F. Russell, 4 September 1925, RAC, RG 1.1, series 100, box 20, folder 169.

Letter from S. Gunn to F. F. Russell, 23 October 1925, RAC, RG 1.1, series 100, box 20, folder 169.

Letter from S. Gunn to F. F. Russell, 16 July 1926, RAC, RG 1.1, series 100, box 20, folder 169.

Letter from S. Gunn to F. F. Russell, 30 August 1926, RAC, RG 1.1, series 100, box 20, folder 170 (1926).

Letter from Dr Heiser, 26 March 1927, RAC, RG 1.1, series 100, box 20, folder 171.

Letter from F. F. Russell to Strode, 25 April 1928, RAC, RG 1.1, series 100, box 20, folder 172.

Letter from L. Rajchman to G. K. Strode, 16 March 1928, RAC, RG 1.1, series 100, box 20, folder 172 (1928).

Letter from L. Rajchman to G. K. Strode, 16 March 1928, RG 1.1, series 100, box 21, folder 173 (June–December, 1928).

Letter from Strode to F. F. Russell, 22 May 1929, RAC, RG 1.1, series 100, box 21, folder 175 (1930).

Letter from W. H. Howell to F. F. Russell, 4 June 1930, RG 1.1, series 100, box 21, folder 175 (1930).

Letter from L. Rajchman to F. F. Russell, 17 June 1932, RAC, RG 1.1, series 100, box 21, folder 176 (1931–2).

Letter from Frank G. Boudreau to G. K. Strode, 5 February 1931, RAC, RG 1.1, series 100, box 21, folder 176 (1931–2).

Letter from Boudreau to F. F. Russell, 21 August 1933, RAC, RG 1.1, series 100, box 21, folder 177.

Letter and memorandum from Boudreau to G. K. Strode, 8 November 1933, RAC, RG 1.1, series 100, box 21, folder 177.

Letter No. 387 from G. K. Strode to F. F. Russell, RAC. RG 1.1, series 100, box 21, folder 177 (1933).

Letter from S. Deutschman to G. K. Strode, 6 April 1942, RAC, RG 1.1, series 100, box 22, folder 182 (1942–4).

'Memorandum of the Medical Director to the Members of the Health Committee' Issued by Selskar Gunn to the Rockefeller Foundation Office, November 1922, RAC, RG 1.1, series 100, box 20, folder 165.

Memorandum by S. Gunn, RAC, RG 1.1, series 100, box 20, folder 170 (1926).

Minutes 1922–34. RG 1.1, series 100, box 20, folder 164.

'Note on Grants of the Rockefeller Foundation to the Health Organization of the League of Nations', RAC, RG1.1. Series 100, Box 21, Folder 175.

'Provisional Outline of Topics for Collective Study of Vital Statistics' , RAC, RG 1.1, series 100, box 20, folder 168 (1924).

Rajchman, L., *The League of Nations Health Organisation: What it is and How it Works*, 18 November 1921, RAC, RG 1.1, series 100, box 20, folder 165.

—, 'Report on the Epidemic Situation in Eastern Europe' (18 February 1922), RAC, RG 1.1, series 100, box 20, folder 165.

—, 'Review of the Experience of the Health Organisation of the League of Nations with the System of Interchange of Public Health Personnel', RAC, RG 1.1, series 100, box 20, folder 172 (1928).

—, and J. Monnet, RAC, RG 1.1, series 100, box 22, folder 181 (1938–41).

Report by Professor Léon Bernard on behalf of the Sub-Committee appointed to examine the French Government Proposal for 'The Creation of an International School of Advanced Health Studies at Paris', RG 6.1, series 1.1, box 38, folder 466 (1930).

'Schools of Public Health 1930', RG 6.1, series 1.1, box 38, folder 471 (1930–8).

'Schools of Public Health 1930. Subjects for Teaching ... ', Report from Strode to F. Russell, RG 1.1, series 100, box 21, folder 175 (1930).

Strode, G. K., *Memorandum on The Health Organization of the League of Nations and the Relationship thereto of the International Health Division of the Rockefeller Foundation.* Typewritten, 37 pages, 10 July 1928, RG 1.1, series 100, box 22, folder 184, League of Nations Health Section Reports (1926–34).

—, Semi-Annual Report 1 January – 30 June 1936, Paris Office-IHD, vol. 1., RG 5, series 1, Correspondence, subseries 2 Projects, box 273, folder 2899.

—, 'League of Nations-Health Organisation', Annual report for 1936. Paris Office-IHD, Section 1, RAC, RG 5, series 1. Correspondence, subseries 2 Projects, box 273, folder 2902.

Zinsser, H., *Report on Journey to Russia as epidemic Commissioner of Hygienic Section, LoN, from June 11th to July 20th, 1923*, RG 1.1, series 100, box 22, folder 183, LoN Health Section, Reports (1922–5).

Printed Primary Sources

Annual Report of the Health Organisation for 1925 (Geneva: League of Nations Health Organisation, 1926) C.H. 442.

Biraud, Y., 'L'Organisation d'Hygiène de la Société des Nations et son Service de Renseignements Épidémiologiques', *Revue Médicale Française* (1936), pp. 223–32.

Blankenstein, H. van, *L'Organisation d'Hygiène de la Société des Nations* (Purmerend: J. Musses, 1934).

Blayac, P., *L'Organisation d'Hygiène de la Société des Nations* (Montpellier: Coulet, 1932).

Compte rendu des debats du Congrès international de Bruxelles; session de 1856 (Bruxelles, 1856).

Congrès International de Bienfaisance de Bruxelles. Session 1856 (Bruxelles: Librairie August/December, 1857).

Eppstein, J., *Ten Years' Life of the League of Nations – a History of the Origins of the League and of its Development from 1919 to 1929*, 'Introduction' by the Right Hon. Viscount Cecil of Chelwood and 'Epilogue' by G. Murray (London: May Fair Press, 1929).

European Health Conference held in Warsaw from March 20th to 28th 1922 (Lausanne: League of Nations, 1922).

'Expediture to be met in 1938 out of the revenue of the Rockefeller Library Endowment Fund', *League of Nations Official Journal* (October 1937).

Fodéré, F. E., 'Lazaret', in *Dechambre, Amédée* (dir.) *Dictionnaire encyclopédique des sciences médicales* (Paris: G. Masson and P. Asselin, 1876).

Food Rationing and Supply, 1943/44 (Geneva: League of Nations, 1942).

Fosdick, R. B., 'La Fondation Rockefeller', *Revue de l'oeuvre accomplie en 1936* (New York, 1937).

Greaves, H. R. G., *The League Committees and World Order: A Study of the Permanent Expert Committees of the League of Nations as an Instrument of International Government* (London: Oxford University Press, 1931).

Guide des Archives de la Société des Nations: 1919–1946 (Geneva: Société des Nations, 1946).

Harris, H. W., *What the League of Nations Is* (London: G. Allen & Unwin Ltd, 1925).

Howard-Ellis, C., *The Origin, Structure and Working of the League of Nations* (London: G. Allen & Unwin Ltd, 1928).

Hutt, C. W., *International Hygiene* (London: Methuen & Co., 1927).

International Health Yearbook/Annuaire sanitaire international, Geneva, League of Nations, 6 vols. (1924–30).

Lacaisse, R., *La Société des Nations et la politique sanitaire international* (Lille: Douviez-Bataille, 1925).

—, *L'hygiène international et la Société des Nations* (Paris: Mouvement Sanitaire, 1926).

L'Organisation d'Hygiène de la Société des Nations (Geneva: Socuiété des Nations, 1923).

League of Nations. Information Section. The Health Organization of the League of Nations (Geneva, 1923), 39 pages.

—, *The Health Organization of the League of Nations.* (Geneva, 1926), 48 pages.

—, *The Health Organization of the League of Nations* (Geneva, 1928), 48 pages.

—, *The Health Organization of the League of Nations* (Geneva, 1931).

—, *New Technical Efforts towards a Better Nutrition* (Geneva, 1938).

—, *Nutrition Considered in Relation to Public Health and to Economic Conditions* (Geneva, 1935).

—, *The Health Work of the League of Nations: Thirty-First Session of the Health Committee.* Supplement to the *Monthly Summary of the League of Nations, Geneva* (January, 1940).

[Lindberg, J.], *Food, Famine and Relief, 1940–1946* (Geneva: League of Nations Financial Section and Economic Intelligence Service, 1946).

Mackenzie, D., *World Co-Operation on Health: Problems of Peace*, 12 series (London: Allen & Unwin, 1938).

Myers, D. P., *Nine Years of the League of Nations, 1920–1928* (Boston, MA: World Peace Foundation Pamphlets, 1929).

Negotiations with the Rockefeller Foundation. *League of Nations Official Journal*, November 1922.

Planelles, L., *Juicio critico de la Conferencia Sanitaria Internacional de Viena. Prefacio*: 'Resultados de las conclusiones de la Conferencia Sanitaria Internacional de Constantinopla en 1966' (Madrid: Manuel Minuesa, 1875) p. 12.

Rapport sur l'Organisation et l'Activité de la Séction d'Hygiène pendant le période octobre 1921 – septembre 1922 (Geneva: League of Nations, 1922).

Répertoire des organisations internationes: associations, bureaux, commissions (Geneva: League of Nations, 1936).

Rose, W., 'Epidemic Control in Europe, and the League', *American Review of Reviews*, 46 (1922).

San Martín Alejandro, *La Conferencia Sanitaria Internacional de Dresde* (Madrid: R. Rojas, 1893).

Ten Years of World Co-Operation, 'Foreword' by Sir E. Drummond, Secretariat of the League of Nations (London: Hazell, Watson & Viney, Ltd, 1930).

Vingt-cinq ans d'activité de l'Office International d'Hygiène Publique 1909–1933 (Paris: Office Internationale d'Hygiène Publique, 1933).

Vitta, C., 'Le droit sanitaire international', *Recueil des cours de l'Académie de droit international*, 33 (1930), pp. 545–670.

Wartime Rationing and Consumption (Geneva: League of Nations, 1942).

White, N., *The League of Nations and the Health of the World: Problems of Peace*, second series (London: Humphrey Milford, 1931).

Secondary Sources

Ackerknecht, E. H., 'Anticontagionism between 1821 and 1867', *Bulletin of the History of Medicine*, 22 (1948), pp. 562–93.

Afanasyeva, A., 'Quarantines and Copper Amulets: The Struggle against Cholera in the Kazakh Steppe in the Nineteenth Century', *Jahrbücher für Geschichte Osteuropas*, 61:4 (2013), pp. 489–512.

Andresen, A., W. Hubbard and T. Ryymin (eds), *International and Local Approaches to Health and Health Care* (Oslo: Novus Press, 2010).

—, T. Gronlie, W. Hubbard and T. Ryymin (eds.) *Health Care Systems and Medical Institutions* (Oslo: Novus Press, 2009).

Auciello, N., *Socialismo ed egemonia in Gramsci e Togliatti* (Bari: Edizione De Donato, 1974).

Baick, J. S., 'Cracks in the Foundation: Frederick T. Gates, the Rockefeller Foundation, and the China Medical Board', *Journal of the Gilded Age and Progressive Era*, 3:1 (2004), pp. 59–89.

Balinska, M. A., 'Assistance and Not Mere Relief: The Epidemic Commission of the League of Nations, 1920–1923', in P. Weindling (ed.), *International Health Organisations and Movements 1918–1939* (Cambridge: Cambridge University Press, 1995), pp. 82–108.

Barnett, M., *Empire of Humanity: A History of Humanitarianism* (Ithaca, NY: Cornell University Press, 2011).

—, and T. G. Weiss. (eds), *Humanitarianism in Question: Politics, Power, Ethics* (Ithaca, NY: Cornell University Press, 2008).

Barona, J. L., 'The Rockefeller Foundation, Social Policies and Public Health in Spain, 1920–1939', in K. Petersen, J. Stewart and M. K. Sorensen, *American Foundations and European Welfare States* (Odense: University of Southern Denmark Press, 2013), pp. 33–58.

—, *From Hunger to Malnutrition: The Political Economy of Scientific Knowledge in Europe, 1918–1960* (Brussels: P. I. E. Peter Lang, 2012).

—, 'Public Health Expert and Scientific Authority', in A. Andresen, W. Hubbard and T. Ryymin (eds), *International and Local Approaches to Health and Health Care* (Oslo: Novus Press, 2010), pp. 31–48.

—, *The Problem of Nutrition: Experimental Science, Public Health and Economy in Europe 1914–1945* (Brussels: P. I. E. Peter Lang, 2010).

—, 'In the Name of Health: The "Instituto Nacionald e Higiene Alfonso XIII" and Laboratory Campaigns in Spanish rural áreas and African colonies, 1910–1924', in A. Andresen, T. Gronlie, W. Hubbard and T. Ryymin (eds), *Health Care Systems and Medical Institutions* (Oslo: Novus Press, 2009).

—, 'Nutrition and Health: The International Context During the Interwar Crisis', *Social History of Medicine*, 20:3 (2008), pp. 87–105.

—, and J. Bernabeu, *La Salud y el Estado. El movimiento sanitario internacional y la administración española* (Valencia: PUV, 2008).

—, and S. Cherry (eds), *Health and Medicine in Rural Europe (1850–1945)* (Valencias: SEC-PUV, 2005).

Basch, P. F. 'International Health Before 1900 and The Organization of International Health Since 1900', in *Textbook of International Health* (Oxford: Oxford University Press, 1999), pp. 11–72.

Bashford, A., and C. Hooker (eds), *Contagion: Historical and Cultural Studies* (London: Routledge, 2001).

Beigbeder, Y., M. Nashat, M.-A. Orsini and J. F. Tiercy, *The World Health Organization* (Dordrecht: Martinus Nijhoff Publichers, 1998).

Bender, T., *A Nation Among Nations: America's Place in World History* (New York: Hill & Wang, 2006).

Berliner, H. S., *A System of Scientific Medicine: Philanthropic Foundations in the Flexner Era* (New York: Tavistock, 1985).

Biraud, M., 'Health in Europe: A Survey of the Epidemic and Nutritional Situation', *League of Nations Bulletin of the Health Organisation,* 10 (1943–4), pp. 557–699.

Biswamoy, P., and M. Harrison, *The Social History of Health and Medicine in Colonial India* (London: New York, Routledge, 2009).

Birn, A. E. and E. Fee, 'The Rockefeller Foundation and the International Health Agenda', *The Lancet*, 381 (2013), pp. 1618–19.

Bolling, L. R. and C. Smith, *Private Foreign Aid: US Philanthropy for Relief and Development* (Boulder, CO: Westview Press, 1982).

Bonah, C., 'We Need for Digitalis Preparations What the State has Established for Serum Therapy ... ' from 'Collecting Plants to International Standardization: The Case of Strophantin, 1900–38', in C. Gradmann and J. Simon (eds) *Evaluating and Standardizing Therapeutic Agents, 1890–1950* (New York: Palgrave Macmillan, 2010), pp. 202–28.

Bonastra Tolós, J., *Ciencia, sociedad y planificación territorial en la institución del lazareto* (Barcelona Tesis Doctoral, Publicacions de la Universitat de Barcelona, 2006).

Borowy, I., *Coming to Terms with World Health: The League of Nations Health Organisation 1921–1946* (Frankfurt am Main: Peter Lang, 2009).

— (ed.), *Uneasy Encounters: The Politics of Medicine and Health in China 1900–1937* (Frankfurt am Main: Peter Lang, 2009).

—, and W. D. Gruner (eds), *Facing Illness in Troubled Times: Health in Europe in the Interwar Years 1918–1939* (Frankfurt am Main: Peter Lang, 2005).

Boyce, R., *The Great Interwar Crisis and the Collapse of Globalisation* (Hampshire: Palgrave MacMillan, 2012).

Bremmer, R. H., *American Philanthropy* (Chicago, IL: University Chicago Press, 1988).

Brown, E. R., 'Public Health and Imperialism: Early Rockefeller Programs at Home and Abroad', *American Journal of Public Health*, 66 (1976), p. 903.

—, *Rockefeller Medicine Men: Medicine and Capitalism in America* (Berkeley, CA: University of California Press, 1979).

Bullock, M. B., *An American Transplant: The Rockefeller Foundation and Peking Union Medical College* (Berkeley, CA: University of California Press, 1980).

Canghilhem, G., *Le Normal et le pathologique* (París: Presse Universitaire de France, 1966).

Chapman, T., *The Congress of Vienna: Origins, Processes and Results* (London: Routledge, 1998).

Cockburn, W. C., 'The International Contribution to the Standardization of Biological Substances / W. C. Cockburn. I, Biological Standards and the League of Nations 1921–1946', *Biologicals*, 19:3 (1991), pp. 161–9.

Cohen, W. I., *Empire Without Tears: America's Foreign Relations, 1921–1933* (New York: Alfred A. Knopf, 1987).

Crawford, E., *Nationalism and Internationalism in Science, 1880–1939* (Cambridge: Cambridge University Press, 1992).

Cueto, M., *The Value of Health: A History of the Pan American Health Organization.* University of Rochester Press, 2007.

— (ed.), *Missionaries of Science: the Rockefeller Foundation and Latin America* (Bloomington, IN: Indiana University Press, 1994).

Curti, M., *American Philanthropy Abroad* (New Brunswick, NJ: Rutgers University Press, 1963).

Dallek, R., *Franklin D. Roosevelt and American Foreign Policy, 1932–1945* (Oxford: Oxford University Press, 1995).

Dubin, M., 'The League of Nations Health organization', in P. Weindling (ed.) *International Health Organisations and Movements 1918–1939* (Cambridge: Cambridge University Press, 1995), pp. 56–62.

Dyck, E., and C. Fletcher (eds), *Locating Health: Historical and Anthropological Investigations of Time and Space* (London: Pickering & Chatto, 2010).

Donelli G., and E. Serinaldi, *Della lotta alla malaria alla nascita dell'Istituto di Sanità Pubbica. Il ruolo della Rockefeller Foundation in Italia: 1922–1934* (Roma-Bari: Laterza, 2003).

Dutta, S., 'Plague, Quarantine and Empire: British-Indian Sanitary Strategies in Central Asia, 1897–1907', in P. Biswamoy and M. Harrison, *The Social History of Health and Medicine in Colonial India* (London and New York: Routledge, 2009).

Evans, R., 'Epidemics and Revolutions: Cholera in Nineteenth Century Europe', in P. Slack and T. Ranger (eds), *Epidemics and Ideas: Essays on the Historical Perception of Pestilence* (Oxford: Oxford University Press, 1992), pp. 167–8.

Farley, J., *To Cast Out Disease: A History of the International Health Division of the Rockefeller Foundation (1913–1951)* (Oxford: Oxford University Press, 2004).

Fee E., *Disease and Discovery: A History of the Johns Hopkins School of Hygiene and Public Health, 1916–1939* (Baltimore, MD: Johns Hopkins University Press, 1987).

Fee, E., and R. Acheson (eds), *A History of Education in Public Health* (Oxford: Oxford University Press, 1991).

Fidler, D. P., *International Law and Infectious Diseases* (Oxford: Clarendon Press, 1999).

Fisher, J. C., and D. Amstrong (eds), *A Different Kind of Diplomacy: A Source Book for International Health Volonteers* (San Diego: Plastic Surgery Research Foundation, 1987).

Flora, P. (ed.), *State Formation, Nation-Building and Mass Politics in Europe: The Theory of Stein Rokkan* (Oxford: Oxford University Press, 1996).

Forsythe, D. P., *The Humanitarians: The International Committee of the Red Cross* (Cambridge: Cambridge University Press, 2006).

Fosdick, R. B., *The Story of the Rockefeller Foundation* (London: Odhams Press, 1952).

Friedman, L. J., and M. D. McGarvie (eds), *Charity, Philanthropy, and Civility in American History* (Cambridge: Cambridge University Press, 2003).

Gachelin, G., 'The Construction of a Culture of Standardization at the Institut Pasteur (1885–1900)', in C. Gradmann and J. Simon (eds), *Evaluating and Standardizing Therapeutic Agents, 1890–1950* (New York: Palgrave Macmillan, 2010), pp. 71–88.

Gates, F. T., and R. S. Morison, *Chapters in My Life* (Detroit, MI: Free Press, 1977).

Gemelli, G., J. F. Picard and W. H. Schneider, *Managing Medical Research in Europe: The Role of the Rockefeller Foundation (1920s–1950s)* (Bologna: CLUEB, 1999).

Gesundheit schützen, Risiken erforschen. Wer wir sind, Worauf wir zurückblicken, Was wir leisten (Berlin: Robert Koch-Institut, 2011).

Goodman, N. M., *International Health Organisations and Their Work* (London: Churchill, 1952).

Gradmann, C,. and J. Simon (eds), *Evaluating and Standardizing Therapeutic Agents, 1890–1950* (New York: Palgrave Macmillan, 2010).

Grmek, M. D. (ed.), *Serving the Cause of Public Health, Selected Papers of Andrija Štampar* (Zagreb, 1968).

Harrison, M., *Contagion: How Commerce has Spread Disease* (New Haven, CT: Yale University Press, 2013).

—, 'Disease, Diplomacy and International Commerce: The Origins of International Sanitary Regulation in the Nineteenth Century', *Journal of Global History*, 1 (2006), pp. 197–217.

Hobson, W., *World Health and History* (Bristol : John Wright, 1963).

Howard-Jones, N., *International Public Health between the Two World Wars: The Organisational Problems* (Geneva: WHO, 1978).

Huber, V., 'The Unification of the Globe by Disease? The International Sanitary Conferences on Cholera, 1851–1894', *Historical Journal*, 49:2 (2006), pp. 453–76.

Hutchinson, J. F., *Champions of Charity: War and Rise of the Red Cross.* (Boulder, CO: Westview Press, 1996).

Iriye, A., *Cultural Internationalism and World Order* (Baltimore, MD: Johns Hopkins University Press, 1997).

—, *Global Community: The Role of International Organizations in the Making of the Contemporary World* (Berkeley, CA: University of California Press, 2002).

Kasius, R. V. (ed.), *The Challenge of Facts: Selected Public Health Papers of Edgar Sydenstricker* (New York: Milbank Memorial Fund, 1974).

Keylor, W. R., *The Twentieth Century World: An International History*, 4th edn (New York/Oxford: Oxford University Press, 2001).

Khalid, A., *The Colonial Behemoth: The Sanitary Regulation of Pilgrimage Sites in Northern India, c.1867–1915* (Oxford: University of Oxford, 2008).

—, '"Subordinate" Negotiations: Indigenous Staff, the Colonial State and Public Health', in P. Biswamoy and M. Harrison, *The Social History of Health and Medicine in Colonial India* (London and New York: Routledge, 2009).

Kim, J.-R., '"The Borderline of 'Empire": Japanese Maritime Quarantine in Busan *c.*1876–1910', *Medical History*, 57:2 (2013), pp. 226–48.

Link, E. P., *The Social Ideas of American Phisicians (1776–1976): Studies in the Humanitarian Tradition of Medicine* (London: Associated University Presses, 1992).

Litsion, S., 'Selskar Gunn and China: The Rockefeller Foundation's "Other" Approach to Public Health', *Bulletin of the History of Medicine*, 79 (2005), pp. 295–318.

—, 'The Rockefeller Foundation's Struggle to Correlate Its Existing Medical Program with Public Health Work in China', in I. Borowy (ed.), *Uneasy Encounters: The Politics of Medicine and Health in China 1900–1937* (Frankfurt: Peter Lang, 2009), pp. 177–203.

Livingston, D., *Putting Science in its Place: Geographies of Scientific Knowledge* (Chicago, IL: University of Chicago Press, 2003).

Löwy, I., and P. Zylberman, 'Introduction. Medicine as a Social Instrument: Rockefeller Foundation, 1913–45', *Studies in the History and Philosophy of Biology and Biomedical Sciences*, 31:3 (2000), pp. 365–79.

Manuila, A. (ed.), *EMRO Partner in Health in the Eastern Mediterranean 1949–1989* (Alexandria: World Health Organisation, 1991).

Mateos Jiménez, J. B., 'Actas de las conferencias sanitarias internacionales (1851–1938)', *Revista Española de Salud Pública*, 79:3 (2005), pp. 339–49.

Mateos Jiménez, J. B. ' Nacimiento de la salud internacional', *Revista Española de Salud Pública*, 80:6 (2006), pp. 647–56.

Mazlish, B., and A. Iriye (eds), *The Global History Reader* (New York: Routledge, 2005).

Mazumdar, P. M. H., 'In the Silence of the Laboratory: The League of Nations Standardizes Syphilis Tests', *Social History of Medicine*, 16 (2003), pp. 437–59.

—, 'The State, the Serum Institutes and the League of Nations', in C. Gradmann and J. Simon (eds), *Evaluating and Standardizing Therapeutic Agents, 1890–1950* (New York: Palgrave Macmillan, 2010), pp. 118–38.

Nevins, A., *Study in Power: John D. Rockefeller, Industrialist and Philanthropist*, 2 vols (New York: Charles Scribner's Sons, 1953).

Ninkovich, F., 'The Rockefeller Foundation, China, and Cultural Change', *Journal of American History*, 70 (1984), pp. 799–820.

Northedge, F. S., *The League of Nations: Its Life and Times 1920–1946* (New York: Holmes and Meier, 1986).

Nye, J. S., *Understanding International Conflicts: An Introduction to Theory and History* (New York: Harper Collins, 1993).

One Hundred Years: The Rockefeller Foundation, on www.rockefeller100.org [accessed 3 July 2014].

Page, B. B., and D. A. Valone (eds), *Philanthropic Foundations and the Globalization of Scientific Medicine and Public Health* (Lanham, MD: University Press of America, 2007).

Panisset, U. B., 'Reflexiones sobre la salud como tema internacional', in *Salud Internacional: Un Debated Norte-Sur* (Washington, WA: Organización Panamericana de la Salud, 1992).

Pestre, D., *Science, argent et politique. Un essai d'interprétation* (Paris: INRA Editions, 2003).

Petersen, K., J. Stewart and M. K. Sorensen, *American Foundations and European Welfare States* (Odense: University of Southern Denmark Press, 2013).

Picard, J. F., *La Fondation Rockefeller et la recherche médicale* (París: Presses Universitaires de France, 1999).

Price-Smith, A. T., *The Health of Nations: Infectious Disease, Environmental Change, and Their Effects on National Security and Development* (Cambridge, MA: MIT Press, 2002).

Rabier, C. (ed.), *Fields of Expertise: A Comparative History of Expert Procedures in Paris and London, 1600 to the Present* (Newcastle: Cambridge Scholars Publications, 2007).

Reinisch, J., *The Perils of Peace: The Public Health Crisis in Occupied Germany* (Oxford: Oxford University Press, 2013).

Rodríguez Ocaña, E., 'Foreign Expertise, Political Pragmatism and Professional Elite: The Reockefeller Foundation in Spain, 1919–39', *Studies in History and Philosophy of Biology and Biomedical Sciences*, 31 (2000), pp. 447–61.

Roemer, M. I., '*Internationalism and Public Health*', in *Companion Encyclopaedia of the History of Medicine* (London: Routledge, 1993), pp. 1417–35.

Rosenberg, E. S., *Spreading the American Dream: American Economic and Cultural Expansion, 1890–1945* (New York: Hill and Wang, 1982).

Schaller, M., *The US Crusade in China 1938–1945* (New York: Columbia University Press, 1979).

Sealander, J., *Private Wealth and Public Life: Foundation Philanthropy and the Reshaping of American Social Policy from the Proghressive Era to the New Deal* (Baltimore, MD: Johns Hopkins University Press, 1997).

Secord, J., *Victorian Sensation* (Chicago, IL: University of Chicago Press, 2003).

Ségur-Dupeyron, M. de, *Rapport adessé à son Exc. Ministre du Commerce, chargé de procéder à une enquête sur le divers régimes sanitaires de la Mediterranée* (Paris: Imprimerie Royale, 1834).

Shaplen, R., *Towards the Well Being of Mankind: Fifty Years of the Rockefeller Foundation* (New York: Doubleday & Co., 1964).

Slack, P., and T. Ranger (eds), *Epidemics and Ideas: Essays on the Historical Perception of Pestilence* (Oxford: Oxford University Press, 1992).

Smith, B., *More than Altruism: the Politics of Private Aid* (Princeton, NJ: Princeton University Press, 1992).

Staples, A. L. S., *The Birth of Development: How the World Bank, Food and Agriculture Organization, and World Health Organization Changed the World, 1945–1965* (Ohio, OH: The Kent State University Press, 2006).

Swaan, A. de, *In Care of the State* (Oxford: Polity Press, 1988).

Trentman, F., and F. Just (eds), *Food and Conflict in Europe in the Age of the Two World Wars* (New York: Palgrave, 2006).

Tyrrell, I., *Reforming the World: the Creation of America's Moral Empire* (Princeton, NJ: Princeton University Press, 2010).

Vogel, A., 'Who's Making Global Civil Society? Philanthropy and US Empire in World Society', *British Journal of Sociology*, 57:4 (2006), pp. 635–55.

Vidal Hernández, J. M., *El Llatzeret de Maó, una fortalesa sanitària* (Menorca Institut: Menorquí d'Estudis, 2002).

Walters, F. P., *A History of the League of Nations* (London: Cumberledge, 1952).

Weaver, W., *US Philanthropic Foundations: Their History, Structure, Management, and Record* (New York: Harper and Row, 1967).

Webster, C., *The Congress of Viena 1814–1815* (London: Thames & Hudson, 1963).

Weindling, P., 'Public Health and Political Stabilisation: The Rockefeller Foundation in Central and Eastern Europe between the Two World Wars', *Minerva*, 31 (1993), pp. 253–67.

— (ed.), *International Health Organisations and Movements 1918–1939,* (Cambridge: Cambridge University Press, 1995).

—, 'Philantropy and World Health: The Rockefeller Foundation and the League of Nations Health Organisation', *Minerva*, 35 (1997), p. 13.

Wetherby, A., *The Medical Activists: Humanitarians, Activists, and American Medical Relief to Spain and China, 1936–1949* (PhD Thesis, Oxford University, Oxford, 2014).

World Health Organization Act 1947, on http://www.comlaw.gov.au/Details/C2004C00489 [accessed 18 August 2014].

Zunz, O., *Philanthropy in America: A History* (Princeton, NJ: Princeton University Press, 2011).

NOTES

Introduction

1. R. Boyce, *The Great Interwar Crisis and the Collapse of Globalisation* (Hampshire: Palgrave MacMillan, 2012).
2. A. de Swaan, *In Care of the State* (Oxford: Polity Press, 1988); P. Flora (ed.), *State Formation, Nation-Building and Mass Politics in Europe: The Theory of Stein Rokkan* (Oxford: Oxford University Press, 1996); A. Andresen, W. Hubbard and T. Ryymin (eds), *International and Local Approaches to Health and Health Care* (Oslo: Novus Press, 2010); and I. Borowyand W. D. Gruner (eds), *Facing Illness in Troubled Times: Health in Europe in the Interwar Years 1918–1939* (Frankfurt am Main: Peter Lang, 2005).
3. A. de Swaan, *In Care of the State* (1988); C. Rabier (ed.), *Fields of Expertise: A Comparative History of Expert Procedures in Paris and London, 1600 to the Present* (Newcastle: Cambridge Scholars Publications, 2007); and F. Trentman, and F. Just (eds), *Food and Conflict in Europe in the Age of the Two World Wars* (New York: Palgrave, 2006).
4. E. R. Brown, 'Public Health and Imperialism: Early Rockefeller Programs at Home and Abroad', *American Journal of Public Health*, 66 (1976), pp. 897–903, on p. 903; B. Smith, *More than Altruism: the Politics of Private Aid* (Princeton, NJ: Princeton University Press, 1992); and P. Weindling, 'Public Health and Political Stabilisation: The Rockefeller Foundation in Central and Eastern Europe between the Two World Wars', *Minerva*, 31 (1993), pp. 253–67.
5. A. Vogel, 'Who's Making Global Civil Society: Philanthropy and US Empire in World Society', *British Journal of Sociology*, 57:4 (2006), pp. 635–55, on pp. 638 and 636.
6. E. S. Rosenberg, *Spreading the American Dream: American Economic and Cultural Expansion, 1890–1945* (New York: Hill and Wang, 1982).
7. J. L. Barona, 'Public Health Expert and Scientific Authority', in Andresen, Hubbard and Ryymin (eds), *International and Local Approaches to Health and Health Care*, p. 31–48; and Rabier (ed.), *Fields of Expertise*.
8. H. S. Berliner, *A System of Scientific Medicine: Philanthropic Foundations in the Flexner Era* (New York: Tavistock, 1985); and B. B. Page and D. A. Valone (eds), *Philanthropic Foundations and the Globalization of Scientific Medicine and Public Health* (Lanham, MD: University Press of America, 2007).
9. L. R. Bolling and C. Smith, *Private Foreign Aid: US Philanthropy for Relief and Development* (Boulder, CO: Westview Press, 1982); R. H. Bremmer, *American Philanthropy* (Chicago, IL: University Chicago Press, 1988); M. Curti, *American Philanthropy Abroad* (New Brunswick: Rutgers University Press, 1963); L. J. Friedman, and M. D.

McGarvie (eds), *Charity, Philanthropy, and Civility in American History* (Cambridge: Cambridge University Press, 2003); J. Sealander, *Private Wealth and Public Life: Foundation Philanthropy and the Reshaping of American Social Policy from the Progbressive Era to the New Deal* (Baltimore, MD: Johns Hopkins University Press, 1997); and O. Zunz, *Philanthropy in America: A History* (Princeton, NJ: Princeton University Press, 2011).

10. A. Wetherby, *The Medical Activists: Humanitarians, Activists, and American Medical Relief to Spain and China, 1936–1949* (PhD Thesis, Oxford University, Oxford, 2014).
11. League of Nations(LoN) Archives, 'Report of the Health Committee to the Permanent Committee ... ', A.22.1924.III.

1 International Diplomacy Meets Public Health

1. D. Pestre, *Science, argent et politique. Un essai d'interprétation* (Paris: INRA Editions, 2003).
2. D. Livingston, *Putting Science in its Place: Geographies of Scientific Knowledge* (Chicago, IL: University of Chicago Press, 2003); and J. Secord, *Victorian Sensation* (Chicago, IL: University of Chicago Press, 2003).
3. N. Auciello, *Socialismo ed egemonia in Gramsci e Togliatti* (Bari: Edizione De Donato, 1974); and J. S. Nye, *Understanding International Conflicts: An Introduction to Theory and History* (New York: Harper Collins, 1993).
4. M. Harrison, *Contagion: How Commerce has Spread Disease* (New Haven, CT: Yale University Press, 2013).
5. M. Harrison, 'Disease, Diplomacy and International Commerce: The Origins of International Sanitary Regulation in the Nineteenth Century', *Journal of Global History*, 1 (2006), pp. 197–217.
6. J. L. Barona and J. Bernabeu, *La Salud y el Estado. El movimiento sanitario internacional y la administración española* (Valencia: PUV, 2008).
7. J. L. Barona and S. Cherry (eds), *Health and Medicine in Rural Europe (1850–1945)* (Valencias: SEC-PUV, 2005).
8. J. L. Barona, 'Public Health Expert and Scientific Authority', in A. Andresen, W. Hubbard and T. Ryymin (eds), *International and Local Approaches to Health and Health Care* (Oslo: Novus Press, 2010), pp. 31–48.
9. J. L. Barona, 'In the Name of Health: The "Instituto Nacionald e Higiene Alfonso XIII" and Laboratory Campaigns in Spanish rural áreas and African colonies, 1910–1924', in A. Andresen, T. Gronlie, W. Hubbard and T. Ryymin (eds), *Health Care Systems and Medical Institutions* (Oslo: Novus Press, 2009), pp. 154–69; and *Gesundheit schützen, Risiken erforschen. Wer wir sind, Worauf wir zurückblicken, Was wir leisten* (Berlin: Robert Koch-Institut, 2011).
10. J. Farley, *To Cast Out Disease: A History of the International Health Division of the Rockefeller Foundation (1913–1951)* (Oxford: Oxford University Press, 2004).
11. E. H. Ackerknecht, 'Anticontagionism between 1821 and 1867', *Bulletin of the History of Medicine*, 22 (1948), pp. 562–93.
12. M. Harrison, 'Disease, Diplomacy and International Commerce: The Origins of International Sanitary Regulation in the Nineteenth Century', *Journal of Global History*, 1 (2006), pp. 197–217; and M. Harrison, *Contagion: How Commerce has Spread Disease* (New Haven, CT: Yale University Press, 2013).
13. J. Bonastra Tolós, *Ciencia, sociedad y planificación territorial en la institución del lazareto* (Barcelona Tesis Doctoral, Publicacions de la Universitat de Barcelona, 2006); and J.

M. Vidal Hernández, *El Llatzeret de Maó, una fortalesa sanitària* (Menorca Institut: Menorquí d'Estudis, 2002).

14. Harrison, *Contagion.*
15. Meaningful contributions are: A. Afanasyeva, 'Quarantines and Copper Amulets: The Struggle against Cholera in the Kazakh Steppe in the Nineteenth Century', *Jahrbücher für Geschichte Osteuropas*, 61:4 (2013), pp. 489–512; A. Bashford and C. Hooker (eds), *Contagion: Historical and Cultural Studies* (London: Routledge, 2001); P. Biswamoy and M. Harrison, *The Social History of Health and Medicine in Colonial India* (London: New York, Routledge, 2009); S. Dutta, 'Plague, Quarantine and Empire: British-Indian Sanitary Strategies in Central Asia, 1897–1907', in Biswamoy and Harrison, *The Social History of Health and Medicine*; A. Khalid, *The Colonial Behemoth: The Sanitary Regulation of Pilgrimage Sites in Northern India, c.1867–1915* (Oxford: University of Oxford, 2008); A. Khalid, '"Subordinate" Negotiations: Indigenous Staff, the Colonial State and Public Health', in Biswamoy and Harrison, *The Social History of Health and Medicine*; J.-R.Kim, '"The Borderline of 'Empire": Japanese Maritime Quarantine in Busan *c.*1876–1910', *Medical History*, 57:2 (2013), pp. 226–48; M. Schaller, *The US Crusade in China 1938–1945* (New York: Columbia University Press, 1979); and I. Tyrrell, *Reforming the World: the Creation of America's Moral Empire* (Princeton, NJ: Princeton University Press, 2010).
16. Harrison, *Contagion.*
17. J. Barona and J. Bernabeu, *La Salud y el Estado. El movimiento sanitario internacional y la administración española* (Valencia: PUV, 2008); and Harrison, 'Disease, Diplomacy and International Commerce', pp. 197–217.
18. T. Chapman, *The Congress of Vienna: Origins, Processes and Results* (London: Routledge, 1998); and C. Webster, *The Congress of Viena 1814–1815* (London: Thames & Hudson, 1963).
19. V. Hube, 'The Unification of the Globe by Disease? The International Sanitary Conferences on Cholera, 1851–1894', *Historical Journal*, 49:2 (2006), pp. 453–76.
20. Ackerknecht, 'Anticontagionism'.
21. Harrison, *Contagion.*
22. F. E. Fodéré, 'Lazaret', in *Dechambre, Amédée* (dir.) *Dictionnaire encyclopédique des sciences médicales* (Paris: G. Masson and P. Asselin, 1876).
23. S. M. Alejandro, *La Conferencia Sanitaria Internacional de Dresde* (Madrid: R. Rojas, 1893).
24. M. de Ségur-Dupeyron, *Rapport adessé à son Exc. Ministre du Commerce, chargé de procéder à une enquête sur le divers régimes sanitaires de la Mediterranée* (Paris: Imprimerie Royale, 1834).
25. The most relevant International Sanitary Conferences are listed on Appendix I at the end of this volume.
26. L. Planelles, *Juicio critico de la Conferencia Sanitaria Internacional de Viena. Prefacio:* 'Resultados de las conclusiones de la Conferencia Sanitaria Internacional de Constantinopla en 1966' (Madrid: Manuel Minuesa, 1875) p. 12.
27. Two volumes were published in Brussels in 1856 in French: *Compte rendu des debats du Congrès international de Bruxelles; session de 1856* (Bruxelles, 1856).
28. Two volumes were published in Brussels in 1858 in French under the title *Congrès International de Bienfaissance de Francfort sur-le-Mein.*
29. Attention was paid on spa institutions and other similar institutions. Interest was justified by being 'one of the most effective means of relieving suffering of humanity; and

industrial concept, being the local baths and medicinal waters an industry of considerable returns'. *Congrès International de Bienfaissance de Francfort sur-le-Mein* (Bruxelles: Th. Lesigne, 1858).

30. Signatories of the charter were the following delegates: E. Beco and O. Velghe (Belgium), E. de Salles Guerra and H. de Rocha Lima (Brazil), M. Tolosa Latour and P. Soler (Spain), A. M. Laughlin and R. S. Reynolds Hitt (United States), C. Barrère, J. de Cazotte and E. Ronssin (France), T. Thomson and B. Franklin (United Kingdom), R. Santoliquido and A. Cotta (Italy), H. de Weede (the Netherlands), M. de Cavalho e Vaconcellos (Portugal), Baron Korff (Russia), J. B. Pioda (Switzerland) and I. Neguib and M. A. Ruffer (Egypt).
31. *Vingt-cinq ans d'activité de l'Office International d'Hygiène Publique 1909–1933* (Paris: Office Internationale d'Hygiène Publique, 1933).
32. Annexe. *Status organique de l'Office International d'Hygiène Publique*, Article 4.
33. Letter from L. Rajchman to Wickliffe Rose, 1922, RAC RG 1.1, series 100, box 20, folder 165.
34. M. Barnett, *Empire of Humanity: A History of Humanitarianism* (Ithaca, NY: Cornell University Press, 2011); L. R. Bolling and C. Smith, *Private Foreign Aid: US Philanthropy for Relief and Development* (Boulder, CO: Westview Press, 1982); R. H. Bremmer, *American Philanthropy* (Chicago, IL: University Chicago Press, 1988); M. Curti, *American Philanthropy Abroad* (New Brunswick, NJ: Rutgers University Press, 1963); N. M. Goodman, *International Health Organisations and Their Work* (London: Churchill, 1952); K. Petersen, J. Stewart and M. K. Sorensen, *American Foundations and European Welfare States* (Odense: University of Southern Denmark Press, 2013); A. Wetherby, *The Medical Activists: Humanitarians, Activists, and American Medical Relief to Spain and China, 1936–1949* (PhD Thesis, Oxford University, Oxford, 2014); and O. Zunz, *Philanthropy in America: A History* (Princeton, NJ: Princeton University Press, 2011).
35. R. B. Fosdick, 'La Fondation Rockefeller', *Revue de l'oeuvre accomplie en 1936* (New York, 1937); *One Hundred Years: The Rockefeller Foundation*, on www.rockefeller100.org [accessed 3 July 2014]; A. Nevins, *Study in Power: John D. Rockefeller, Industrialist and Philanthropist*, 2 vols (New York: Charles Scribner's Sons, 1953); and R. Shaplen, *Towards the Well Being of Mankind: Fifty Years of the Rockefeller Foundation* (New York: Doubleday & Co., 1964).
36. A. E. Birn and E. Fee, 'The Rockefeller Foundation and the International Health Agenda', *The Lancet*, 381 (2013), pp. 1618–19, on p. 1618.
37. F. T. Gates and R. S. Morison, *Chapters in My Life* (Detroit, MI: Free Press, 1977).
38. Gates and Morison, *Chapters in My Life*.
39. J. Farley, *To Cast Out Disease: A History of the International Health Division of the Rockefeller Foundation (1913–1951)* (Oxford: Oxford University Press, 2004); and I. Löwy, and P. Zylberman, 'Introduction. Medicine as a Social Instrument: Rockefeller Foundation, 1913–45', *Studies in the History and Philosophy of Biology and Biomedical Sciences*, 31:3 (2000), pp. 365–79.
40. R. B. Fosdick, *The Story of the Rockefeller Foundation* (London: Odhams Press, 1952), p. 9.
41. M. Cueto (ed.), *Missionaries of Science: the Rockefeller Foundation and Latin America* (Bloomington, IN: Indiana University Press, 1994).
42. Fosdick, *The Story of the Rockefeller Foundation*, p. 10.
43. Birn and Fee, 'The Rockefeller Foundation', p. 1618.
44. Fosdick, *The Story of the Rockefeller Foundation*, p. 14.
45. Fosdick, *The Story of the Rockefeller Foundation*, p. 15.
46. I. Borowy (ed.), *Uneasy Encounters: The Politics of Medicine and Health in China*

1900–1937 (Frankfurt am Main: Peter Lang, 2009); S. Litsion, 'Selskar Gunn and China: The Rockefeller Foundation's "Other" Approach to Public Health', *Bulletin of the History of Medicine*, 79 (2005), pp. 295–318; S. Litsios, 'The Rockefeller Foundation's Struggle to Correlate Its Existing Medical Program with Public Health Work in China', in Borowy (ed.), *Uneasy Encounters*, pp. 177–203; F. Ninkovich, 'The Rockefeller Foundation, China, and Cultural Change', *Journal of American History*, 70 (1984), pp. 799–820; and Wetherby, *The Medical Activists*.

47. Fosdick, *The Story of the Rockefeller Foundation*, p. 15.
48. Petersen, Stewart and Sorensen, *American Foundations*, p. 11.
49. Fosdick, *The Story of the Rockefeller Foundation*.
50. *One Hundred Years*, on www.rockefeller100.org.
51. Suggested draft letter from the secretary-general of the League of Nations to the International Health Board of the Rockefeller Foundation. League of Nations Official Journal, November 1922, 1256.
52. Fosdick, 'La Fondation Rockefeller'.
53. G. Gemelli, J. F. Picard and W. H. Schneider, *Managing Medical Research in Europe: The Role of the Rockefeller Foundation (1920s–1950s)* (Bologna: CLUEB, 1999).
54. *Ten Years of World Co-Operation*, 'Foreword' by Sir E. Drummond, Secretariat of the League of Nations (London: Hazell, Watson & Viney, Ltd, 1930), p. 257.
55. *Ten Years of World Co-Operation*, p. 260.
56. J. L. Barona and J. Bernabeu, *La Salud y el Estado. El movimiento sanitario internacional y la administración española* (Valencia: PUV, 2008).
57. J. L. Barona, 'Nutrition and Health: The International Context During the Interwar Crisis', *Social History of Medicine*, 20:3 (2008), pp. 87–105.
58. I. Borowy, *Coming to Terms with World Health: The League of Nations Health Organisation 1921–1946* (Frankfurt am Main: Peter Lang, 2009).
59. *Ten Years of World Co-Operation,* p. 8.
60. See Appendix II – transcript of the *Health Scheme of the League of Nations*.
61. *Ten Years of World Co-Operation*, p. 8–9.
62. *The League of Nations Starts: An Outline by Its Organisers* (London: MacMillan and Co. Ltd, 1920), on https://archive.org/stream/leagueofnationss015671mbp/leagueofnationss015671mbp_djvu.txt [accessed 27 May 2013].
63. *The League of Nations Starts*.
64. *The League of Nations Starts*; and W. Rose, 'Epidemic Control in Europe, and the League', *American Review of Reviews*, 46 (1922), pp. 77–80, on p. 4.
65. G. K. Strode, *Memorandum on The Health Organization of the League of Nations and the Relationship thereto of the International Health Division of the Rockefeller Foundation.* Typewritten, 37 pages, 10 July 1928, RG 1.1, series 100, box 22, folder 184, League of Nations Health Section Reports (1926–34).
66. The enclosed document was the *Health Scheme of the League of Nations (6th draft)* consisting of eight typewritten pages and signed the 12/12/1919 by Rachel Crowdy, Secretary-Gral of the League of Nations, RAC RG 1.1., series 100, box 20, folder 165.
67. Strode, *Memorandum*, pp. 5–6.
68. Rajchman, L., *The League of Nations Health Organisation: What it is and How it Works*, 18 November 1921, RAC, RG 1.1, series 100, box 20, folder 165.
69. Rose, 'Epidemic Control', p. 11.
70. Letter from Eric Drummond to Wickliffe Rose, 2 September 1922, RAC, RG 1.1, series 100, box 20, folder 165.

71. Letter from Wickliffe Rose to Eric Drummond, 14 June 1922, RAC, RG 1.1, series 100, box 20, folder 165.
72. The full text of the agreement is reproduced in Appendix II.
73. Rockefeller Funds for 1922, RAC, RG 1.1, series 100, box 20, folder 165.
74. *League of Nations Starts.*
75. Borowy, *Coming to Terms with World Health.*
76. Memorandum by S. Gunn, RAC, RG 1.1, series 100, box 20, folder 170 (1926).
77. Memorandum by S. Gunn, (1926).
78. Letter from S. Gunn to F. F. Russell, 30 August 1926, RAC, RG 1.1, series 100, box 20, folder 170 (1926).
79. Letter from S. Gunn to F. F. Russell, 30 August 1926.
80. Strode, *Memorandum.*
81. Strode, *Memorandum,* pp. 11–12.
82. Strode, *Memorandum,* p. 12.
83. Strode, *Memorandum,* p. 13.
84. L. Rajchman, 'Review of the Experience of the Health Organisation of the League of Nations with the System of Interchange of Public Health Personnel', RAC, RG 1.1, series 100, box 20, folder 172 (1928).
85. Letter from F. F. Russell to G. K. Strode, 25 April 1928, RAC, RG 1.1, series 100, box 20, folder 172.
86. Letter from Russell to Strode, 25 April 1928.
87. Strode, *Memorandum,* p. 15.
88. Strode, *Memorandum,* pp. 16–17.
89. Strode, *Memorandum,* p. 18.
90. Letter from L. Rajchman to G. K. Strode, 16 March 1928, RAC, RG 1.1, series 100, box 20, folder 172 (1928).
91. Letter from L. Rajchman to G. K. Strode, 16 March 1928.
92. Strode. *Memorandum,* pp. 28–9.
93. Strode. *Memorandum,* p. 32.
94. Strode. *Memorandum,* p. 35.
95. Strode. *Memorandum,* pp. 36–7.
96. Letter from Strode to F. F. Russell, 22 May 1929, RAC, RG 1.1, series 100, box 21, folder 175 (1930).
97. Letter from Strode to F.F. Russell, 22 May 1929; Letter from L. Rajchman to F. F. Russell, 17 June, 1932, RAC, RG 1.1, series 100, box 21, folder 176 (1931–2).
98. Letter from S. Gunn to F. F. Russell, 4 September 1925, RAC, RG 1.1, series 100, box 20, folder 169.
99. Letter from Gunn to Russell, 4 September 1925.
100. Sir George Newman was a public health expert, Quaker, the first Chief Medical Officer to the Ministry of Health in England and an active contributor to the creation of the Far East Bureau in Singapore.
101. Letter from Rajchman to Strode, 16 March.
102. Letter from Rajchman to Strode, 16 March 1928, p. 4–5.
103. Letter from Rajchman to Strode, 16 March 1928, p. 4–5.
104. Letter from Boudreau to F. F. Russell, 21 August 1933, RAC, RG 1.1, series 100, box 21, folder 177.
105. Letter and memorandum from Boudreau to G. K. Strode, 8 November 1933, RAC, RG 1.1, series 100, box 21, folder 177.

106. Letter and memorandum from Boudreau to Strode, 8 November 1933.
107. Letter from Boudreau to Russell, RAC, RG 1.1, series 100, box 21, folder 177 (1933).
108. Letter and memorandum from Boudreau to Strode, 8 November 1933.
109. Letter and memorandum from Boudreau to Strode, 8 November 1933.
110. Letter and memorandum from Boudreau to Strode, 8 November 1933.
111. Letter and memorandum from Boudreau to Strode, 8 November 1933.
112. Letter and memorandum from Boudreau to Strode, 8 November 1933.
113. Letter and memorandum from Boudreau to Strode, 8 November 1933.
114. Letter and memorandum from Boudreau to Strode, 8 November 1933.
115. Letter and memorandum from Boudreau to Strode, 8 November 1933.
116. Letter and memorandum from Boudreau to Strode, 8 November 1933.
117. Letter and memorandum from Boudreau to Strode, 8 November 1933.
118. Letter and memorandum from Boudreau to Strode, 8 November 1933.
119. Letter No. 387 from G. K. Strode to F.F. Russell, RAC. RG 1.1, series 100, box 21, folder 177 (1933).
120. Letter No. 387 from Strode to Russell (1933).
121. G. K. Strode, Semi-Annual Report 1 January–30 June 1936, Paris Office-IHD, vol. 1., RG 5, series 1, Correspondence, subseries 2 Projects, box 273, folder 2899.
122. Strode, Semi-Annual Report 1 January – 30 June 1936, pp. 6–7.

2 The First Great Intervention: Epidemics and Famine in Eastern Europe

1. *European Health Conference held in Warsaw from March 20th to 28th 1922* (Lausanne: League of Nations, 1922).
2. 'Dr Syssin's Summary of General Situation and Prospects for Working with League of Nations. Report of the Sanitary Epidemiologic Section of the Commissariat of Public Health Referring to Struggle with Cholera', RAC, RG 1.1, series 100, box 22, folder 183 (1922–5).
3. *Feldshers* were traditional healers providing primary, obstetrical and surgical health care in rural areas of Russia.
4. 'Dr Syssin's Summary' (1921), pp. 4–5.
5. 'Dr Syssin's Summary' (1921), p. 5.
6. 'Dr Syssin's Summary' (1921), p. 6; and International Health Conference (London, 1920), Minutes, 10/51/1–20/51/8.
7. 'Dr Syssin's Summary' (1921), p. 6; and International Health Conference (1920), Minutes, 10/51/1–20/51/8.
8. 'Dr Syssin's Summary' (1921), p. 6; and International Health Conference (1920), Minutes, 10/51/1–20/51/8.
9. M. A. Balinska, 'Assistance and Not Mere Relief: The Epidemic Commission of the League of Nations, 1920–1923', in P. Weindling (ed.), *International Health Organisations and Movements 1918–1939* (Cambridge: Cambridge University Press, 1995), pp. 82–108.
10. *European Health Conference held in Warsaw* (1922).
11. *European Health Conference held in Warsaw* (1922).
12. *European Health Conference held in Warsaw* (1922).
13. *European Health Conference held in Warsaw* (1922).
14. W. Rose, 'Epidemic Control in Europe, and the League', *American Review of Reviews*, 46 (1922).

15. L. Rajchman, 'Report on the Epidemic Situation in Eastern Europe' (18 February 1922), RAC, RG 1.1, series 100, box 20, folder 165.
16. Rajchman, 'Report on the Epidemic Situation' (February 1922).
17. Rajchman, 'Report on the Epidemic Situation' (February 1922).
18. Rajchman, 'Report on the Epidemic Situation' (February 1922).
19. Rajchman, 'Report on the Epidemic Situation' (February 1922).
20. L. Rajchman, 'Report on the Epidemic Situation in Eastern Europe' (18 February 1922), RAC, RG 1.1, series 100, box 20, folder 165.
21. Rajchman, 'Report on the Epidemic Situation' (February 1922), p. 2.
22. League of Nations Information Section, *The Health Organization of the League of Nations* (Geneva, 1931), p. 4.
23. L. Rajchman, *The League of Nations Health Organisation: What it is and How it Works*, 18 November 1921, RAC, RG 1.1, series 100, box 20, folder 165.
24. Rajchman, *The League of Nations Health Organisation*.
25. W. Rose, 'Epidemic Control in Europe, and the League', *American Review of Reviews*, 46 (1922).
26. Rose, 'Epidemic Control in Europe'.
27. Rose, 'Epidemic Control in Europe', p. 5.
28. Rose, 'Epidemic Control in Europe', p. 4.
29. H. Zinsser, *Report on Journey to Russia as epidemic Commissioner of Hygienic Section, LoN, from June 11th to July 20th, 1923*, RG 1.1, series 100, box 22, folder 183, LoN Health Section, Reports (1922–5).
30. Zinsser, *Report on Journey to Russia*, p. 2.
31. Zinsser, *Report on Journey to Russia*, p. 4.
32. Zinsser, *Report on Journey to Russia*, p. 11.
33. Zinsser, *Report on Journey to Russia*, p. 11.
34. Zinsser, *Report on Journey to Russia*, p. 15.
35. Zinsser, *Report on Journey to Russia*, p. 18.
36. Zinsser, *Report on Journey to Russia*, pp. 22–3.

3 The Extension of the Collaborative Programme

1. *Ten Years of World Co-Operation*, 'Foreword' by Sir E. Drummond, Secretariat of the League of Nations (London: Hazell, Watson & Viney, Ltd, 1930), p. 242.
2. *League of Nations. Information Section. The Health Organization of the League of Nations* (Geneva, 1923), p. 18.
3. L. Rajchman, *The League of Nations Health Organisation: What it is and How it Works*, 18 November 1921, RAC, RG 1.1, series 100, box 20, folder 165.
4. See Appendix III 'Articles of the Agreement Between the League of Nations Health Organization and the International Health Board of the Rockefeller Foundation'.
5. 'Grant for the Maintenance of a System of Interchange of Public Health Personnel on an International Scale', RAC, RG1.1. Series 100, Box 21, Folder 175 (1930), p. 1.
6. W. Rose, 'Epidemic Control in Europe, and the League', *American Review of Reviews*, 46 (1922), p. 7.
7. I. Borowy, *Coming to Terms with World Health: The League of Nations Health Organisation 1921–1946* (Frankfurt am Main: Peter Lang, 2009), p. 192.
8. L. Rajchman, 'Review of the Experience of the Health Organisation of the League of Nations with the System of Interchange of Public Health Personnel', RAC, RG 1.1,

series 100, box 20, folder 172 (1928).

9. Meeting of Directors of Schools of Public Health in Paris, 20 May 1930, RAC, RG 6.1, series 1.1, box 38, folder 471.
10. Letter from S. Gunn to F. F. Russell, 12 October 1923, RAC, RG 1.1, series 100, box 20, folder 166.
11. Letter from S. Gunn to F. F. Russell, 14 February 1924, RAC, RG 1.1, series 100, box 20, folder 167.
12. Letter from F. F. Russell to S. Gunn, 13 March 1924, RAC, RG 1.1, series 100, box 20, folder 167.
13. Letter from F. F. Russell to S. Gunn, 15 April 1924, RAC, RG 1.1, series 100, box 20, folder 167.
14. Letter from L. Rajchman to S. Gunn, 25 September 1924, RAC, RG 1.1, series 100, box 20, folder 168.
15. Rajchman 'Review of the Experience of the Health' (1928).
16. Letter from D. B. Wilson (Ministerio de Instrucción y Salubridad Públicas) to F. F. Russell, 15 June 1925, RAC, RG 1.1, series 100, box 20, folder 169.
17. Letter from Wilson to Russell, 15 June 1925.
18. Letter from S. Gunn to F. F. Russell, 23 October 1925, RAC, RG 1.1, series 100, box 20, folder 169.
19. Letter from Gunn to Russell, 23 October 1925.
20. Letter from S. Gunn to F. F. Russell, 16 July 1926, RAC, RG 1.1, series 100, box 20, folder 169.
21. Letter from Gunn to Russell, 16 July 1926.
22. Letter from Gunn to Russell, 16 July 1926.
23. Rajchman, 'Review of the Experience of the Health' (1927), p. 7.
24. *Ten Years of World Co-Operation*, p. 243.
25. Rajchman, 'Review of the Experience of the Health' (1927), p. 1.
26. 'Grant for the Maintenance of a System', p. 2.
27. Rajchman, 'Review of the Experience of the Health' (1927), p. 4–5.
28. Rajchman, 'Review of the Experience of the Health' (1927), p. 5.
29. 'Grant for the Maintenance of a System', p. 3.
30. 'Grant for the Maintenance of a System', p. 3.
31. A. Lutrario, President of the Malaria Commission, Confidential Report presented to the RF on the Work of the Malaria Commission, March 1925, RAC, RG 1.1, series 100, box 20, folder 169.
32. S. Gunn Report on the visit of the Malaria Commission to the United States during 1925 and 1926, RAC, RG 1.1, series 100, box 20, folder 170.
33. Rajchman, 'Review of the Experience of the Health' (1927), p. 5.
34. 'Grant for the Maintenance of a System', p. 5.
35. *Annual Report of the Health Organisation for 1925* (Geneva: League of Nations Health Organisation, 1926), C. H. 442.
36. 'Schools of Public Health 1930', RG 6.1, series 1.1, box 38, folder 471 (1930–8).
37. J. L. Barona, 'Public Health Expert and Scientific Authority', in A. Andresen, W. Hubbard and T. Ryymin (eds), *International and Local Approaches to Health and Health Care* (Oslo: Novus Press, 2010), pp. 31–48.
38. 'Schools of Public Health 1930. Subjects for Teaching ... ', Report from Strode to F. Russell, RG 1.1, series 100, box 21, folder 175 (1930).
39. J. L. Barona, 'The European Conference of Rural Health (1930, 1931)', in J. L. Barona

and S. Cherry (eds), *Health and Medicine in Rural Europe (1850–1945)* (Valencia: SEC-PUV, 2005); and 'Schools of Public Health 1930. Subjects for Teaching'.
40. 'Grant for the Maintenance of a System', p. 5.
41. Letter from Frank G. Boudreau to G. K. Strode, 5 February 1931, RAC, RG 1.1, series 100, box 21, folder 176 (1931–2).
42. Letter from Boudreau to Strode, 5 February 1931, RAC, RG 1.1, series 100, box 21, folder 176 (1931–2), pp. 4–5.
43. Letter from Boudreau to Strode, 5 February 1931, pp. 4–5.
44. Letter from Boudreau to Strode, 5 February 1931, p. 5.
45. 'Schools of Public Health 1930. Subjects for Teaching'.
46. 'Schools of Public Health 1930' (1930–8).
47. 'Schools of Public Health 1930' (1930–8).
48. 'Schools of Public Health 1930. Subjects for Teaching'.
49. 'Schools of Public Health 1930. Subjects for Teaching'.
50. Barona 'Public Health Expert'.
51. Letter from W. H. Howell to F. Russell, 4 June 1930. RG 1.1, series 100, box 21, folder 175 (1930).
52. Letter from Howell to Russell, 4 June 1930, p. 3.
53. Letter from Howell to Russell, 4 June 1930, pp. 3–4.
54. Letter from L. Rajchman to F. F. Russell, 17 June 1932, RAC, RG 1.1, series 100, box 21, folder 176 (1931–2).
55. Report by Professor Léon Bernard on behalf of the Sub-Committee appointed to examine the French Government Proposal for 'The Creation of an International School of Advanced Health Studies at Paris', RG 6.1, series 1.1, box 38, folder 466 (1930).
56. L. Rajchman and J. Monnet, RAC, RG 1.1, series 100, box 22, folder 181 (1938–41).
57. Letter from S. Deutschman to G. K. Strode, 6 April 1942, RAC, RG 1.1, series 100, box 22, folder 182 (1942–4).
58. Letter from Deutschman to Strode, 6 April 1942.
59. 'Note on Grants of the Rockefeller Foundation to the Health Organization of the League of Nations', RAC, RG1.1. Series 100, Box 21, Folder 175.
60. 'Epidemiological Intelligence Service', RAC, RG 1.1, series 100, box 20, folder 165.
61. 'Epidemiological Intelligence Service'.
62. 'Epidemiological Intelligence Service'.
63. Letter from E. Drummond to W. Rose, 2 September 1922, RAC, RG 1.1, series 100, box 20, folder 165.
64. Letter from Drummond to Rose, 2 September 1922.
65. This is a direct reference against the implication of the IHD of the Rockefeller Foundation.
66. Letter from G. Buchanan to T. Madsen, 27 July 1922. RAC, RG 1.1, series 100, box 20, folder 165, p. 5.
67. Letter from Buchanan to Madsen, 27 July 1922, p. 5.
68. Letter from S. Gunn to F. F. Russell, 28 August 1925, RAC RG 1.1, series 100, box 20, folder 169.
69. W. Rose, 'Epidemic Control in Europe, and the League', *American Review of Reviews*, 46 (1922), p. 9.
70. Letter from Buchanan to Madsen, 27 July 1922.
71. Letter from Buchanan to Madsen, 27 July 1922.
72. Letter from Drummond to Rose, 2 September 1922.
73. 'Memorandum of the Medical Director to the Members of the Health Committee'

Issued by Selskar Gunn to the Rockefeller Foundation Office, November 1922, RAC, RG 1.1, series 100, box 20, folder 165.

74. 'Memorandum of the Medical Director', November 1922.
75. Minutes of the International Health Board of the Rockefeller Foundation (1922), RAC, RG 1.1, series 100, box 20, folder 164.
76. See R. V. Kasius (ed.), *The Challenge of Facts: Selected Public Health Papers of Edgar Sydenstricker* (New York: Milbank Memorial Fund, 1974).
77. J. Eppstein, *Ten Years' Life of the League of Nations – a History of the Origins of the League and of its Development from 1919 to 1929*, 'Introduction' by the Right Hon. Viscount Cecil of Chelwood and 'Epilogue' by G. Murray (London: May Fair Press, 1929); and *Ten Years of World Co-Operation*, 'Foreword' by Sir E. Drummond, Secretariat of the League of Nations (London: Hazell, Watson & Viney, Ltd, 1930).
78. *Ten Years of World Co-Operation*, p. 240.
79. 'Provisional Outline of Topics for Collective Study of Vital Statistics', RAC, RG 1.1, series 100, box 20, folder 168 (1924).
80. 'Grant for Training in Methods of Vital and Public Health Statistics', RG 1.1, series 100, box 21, folder 174 (1929), p. 5.
81. 'Grant for Training', p. 1.
82. Letter from Eichel to Russell, 30 May 1924, RAC, RG 1.1, series 100, box 20, folder 167.
83. Letter from Eichel to Russell, 30 May 1924.
84. Letter from F. M. Read answered to Eichel, 20 June 1924, RG 1.1, series 100, box 20, folder 167.
85. Letter from F. F. Russell to S. Gunn, 15 April 1924, RAC, RG 1.1, series 100, box 20, folder 167.
86. Letter from S. Gunn to L. Rajchman, 2 September 1924, RAC, RG 1.1, series 100, box 20, folder 168.
87. Letter from L. Rajchman to S. Gunn, 3 September 1924, RAC, RG 1.1, series 100, box 20, folder 168.
88. Letter from Rajchman to Gunn, 3 September 1924.
89. Letter from L. Rajchman to S. Gunn, 8 September 1924, RAC, RG 1.1, series 100, box 20, folder 168.
90. 'Note on Grants of the Rockefeller Foundation', p. 4.
91. Annual Report of the Health Organization, 1925, C.H. 442 (A.17.1926.III).
92. Letter from F. F. Russell to S. Gunn, 13 March 1924, RAC, RG 1.1, series 100, box 20, folder 167.
93. 'Grant by the Rockefeller Foundation for the Establishment and Upkeep of the Health Organisation's Eastern Bureau at Singapore', RAC, RG1.1. Series 100, Box 21, Folder 175 (1930), p. 1.
94. 'Grant by the Rockefeller Foundation', p. 1.
95. Letter from F. F. Russell to S. Gunn, 11 October, 1924, RAC, RG 1.1, series 100, box 20, folder 168.
96. Letter of N. White to F. F. Russell, 20 November 1924, RAC, RG 1.1, series 100, box 20, folder 168.
97. Service of Epidemiological Intelligence, Official Statistical Records, RAC, RG 1.1, series 100, box 20, folder 168 (1924).
98. RAC, RG 1.1, series 100, box 20, folder 168 (1924).
99. 'Grant by the Rockefeller Foundation', p. 2.

100. Those countries were British India, British North Borneo, Ceylon, China, Federated Malay States, French Indo-China, Hong Kong, Japan, the Netherlands East Indies, Philippine Islands, Sian and the Straits Settlements.
101. Letter from L. Rajchman to S. Gunn, 14 February 1925, RAC, RG 1.1, series 100, box 20, folder 169.
102. Letter from Dr Heiser, 26 March 1927, RAC, RG 1.1, series 100, box 20, folder 171.
103. 'Grant by the Rockefeller Foundation', p. 3.
104. 'Grant by the Rockefeller Foundation', p. 6.
105. 'Grant by the Rockefeller Foundation', p. 7.
106. Letter from L. Rajchman to G. K. Strode, 16 March 1928, RAC, RG 1.1, series 100, box 20, folder 172 (1928).
107. Letter from L. Rajchman to G. K. Strode, 16 March 1928, RG 1.1, series 100, box 21, folder 173 (June–December, 1928).
108. 'Grant by the Rockefeller Foundation', p. 7.
109. 'Grant by the Rockefeller Foundation', p. 6.
110. RG 1.1, series 100, box 20, folder 164 (Minutes 1922–34) and RG 1.1, series 100, box 20, folder 171 (1927).
111. Minutes of the International Health Division, RG 1.1, series 100, box 20, folder 171 (1927).
112. 'Grant by the Rockefeller Foundation for the Support of a Centre of Public Health Documentation', RAC, RG1.1. Series 100, Box 21, Folder 175 (1930).
113. 'Grant by the Rockefeller Foundation for the Support', p. 2.
114. 'Grant by the Rockefeller Foundation for the Support', p. 3.
115. 'Grant by the Rockefeller Foundation for the Support', p. 4.
116. C. Gradmann and J. Simon (eds) *Evaluating and Standardizing Therapeutic Agents, 1890–1950* (New York: Palgrave Macmillan, 2010), pp. 202–28.
117. C. Bonah, 'We Need for Digitalis Preparations What the State has Established for Serumtherapy ... ', from 'Collecting Plants to International Standardization: The Case of Strophantin, 1900–38', in Gradmann and Simon (eds), *Evaluating and Standardizing Therapeutic Agents*, pp. 202–28.
118. G. Canghilhem, *Le Normal et le pathologique* (París: Presse Universitaire de France, 1966).
119. Gradmann and Simon (eds), *Evaluating and Standardizing Therapeutic Agents.*
120. Gradmann and Simon (eds), *Evaluating and Standardizing Therapeutic Agents.*
121. Gradmann and Simon (eds), *Evaluating and Standardizing Therapeutic Agents*, p. 7.
122. G. Gachelin, 'The Construction of a Culture of Standardization at the Institut Pasteur (1885–1900)', in Gradmann and Simon (eds), *Evaluating and Standardizing Therapeutic Agents*, pp. 71–88.
123. International Conference on the Standardisation of Sera and Serological Tests (London, 1921), League of Nations Archives, C.533.M.378.1921.III.
124. International Conference on the Standardisation (London, 1921).
125. International Conference on the Standardisation (London, 1921).
126. W. Rose, 'Epidemic Control in Europe, and the League', *American Review of Reviews*, 46 (1922), p. 8.
127. International Conference on the Standardisation (London, 1921).
128. International Conference on the Standardisation (London, 1921).
129. In 1921 the Conference on the Standardization of será and serological tests took place in London, and the second was held in Paris in 1922: International Conference on the Standardisation of Sera and Serological Tests (second) (Paris, 1922), League of Nations

Archives, C.H./S.S. 1 – C.H./S.S. 32.

130. Technical Conference for Consideration of Certain Methods of Biological Standardisation (Edinburgh, 1923), League of Nations Archives, C.H./B. 1– C.H./B. 3; and Technical Laboratory Conference on the Serodiagnosis of Syphilis (Copenhagen, 1923), League of Nations Archives, C.5.M.1924.III.
131. *IHD League of Nations-Permanent Standardization Commission* (1934–38), RAC, RG 6.1, series 1.1, box 38, folder 468.
132. *IHD League of Nations* (1934–38), folder 468.
133. P. M. H. Mazumdar, 'The State, the Serum Institutes and the League of Nations', in Gradmann and Simon (eds), *Evaluating and Standardizing Therapeutic Agents*, pp. 118–38. See also: P. M. H. Mazumdar, 'In the Silence of the Laboratory: The League of Nations Standardizes Syphilis Tests', *Social History of Medicine*, 16 (2003), pp. 437–59.
134. Report to the Council on the Work of the Twenty-Fourth HC Session, February 1937, C.148.M.96.1937.III, pp. 11–12.
135. J. L. Barona, *The Problem of Nutrition: Experimental Science, Public Health and Economy in Europe 1914–1945* (Brussels: P. I. E. Peter Lang, 2010).
136. Barona, *The Problem of Nutrition*.
137. Barona, *The Problem of Nutrition*.
138. J. L. Barona, *From Hunger to Malnutrition: The Political Economy of Scientific Knowledge in Europe, 1918–1960* (Brussels: P. I. E. Peter Lang, 2012).
139. *Wartime Rationing and Consumption* (Geneva: League of Nations, 1942).
140. [J. Lindberg], *Food, Famine and Relief, 1940–1946* (Geneva: League of Nations Financial Section and Economic Intelligence Service, 1946).
141. *Wartime Rationing and Consumption*.
142. *Wartime Rationing and Consumption*, p. 2.
143. [Lindberg] *Food, Famine and Relief*.
144. Appendix 'Legal Food Rations by Countries, 1940–1945', in [Lindberg] *Food, Famine and Relief*, pp. 121–59.
145. [Lindberg] *Food, Famine and Relief*, p. 3.
146. [Lindberg] *Food, Famine and Relief*, p. 4.

4 International Health and the End of the League of Nations: Gautier's Evaluation

1. I. Borowy, *Coming to Terms with World Health: The League of Nations Health Organisation, 1921–1946* (Frankfurt am Main: Peter Lang, 2009), p. 427.
2. Borowy 2009, p. 427.
3. R. Gautier, Report on 'International Health of the Future', RAC, RG 1.1, series 100, box 22, folder 182 (1942–4), pp. 1–11, on p. 1.
4. Gautier 'International Health', p. 1.
5. This definition contributed by Gautier in his report became the more popular worldwide extended definition of health associated to the World Health Organization sanitary ideology. Something that shows the influence of the Swiss public health expert in the making of the WHO. Gautier 'International Health', p. 1.
6. Gautier 'International Health', p. 3.
7. Gautier 'International Health', p. 3.
8. Gautier 'International Health', p. 4.

9. Gautier 'International Health', p. 5.
10. J. L. Barona, *From Hunger to Malnutrition: The Political Economy of Scientific Knowledge in Europe, 1918–1960* (Brussels: P. I. E. Peter Lang, 2012).
11. Gautier 'International Health', p. 5.
12. Gautier 'International Health', p. 6.
13. Gautier 'International Health', p. 6.
14. Gautier 'International Health', p. 8.
15. Gautier 'International Health', p. 8.
16. Gautier, 'International Health', p. 9.
17. Gautier 'International Health', p. 10.
18. *World Health Organization Act 1947*, on http://www.comlaw.gov.au/Details/C2004C00489 [accessed 18 August 2014].

5 Some General Conclusions

1. G. K. Strode, 'League of Nations-Health Organisation', Annual report for 1936. Paris Office-IHD, Section 1, RAC, RG 5, series 1. Correspondence, Subseries 2 Projects, box 273, folder 2902.
2. Strode, 'League of Nations-Health Organisation', Annual report for 1936.
3. Strode, 'League of Nations-Health Organisation', Annual report for 1936.
4. Strode, 'League of Nations-Health Organisation', Annual report for 1936.

Appendix 1: International Sanitary Conferences, Commissions and Boards, Previous to the League of Nations (1920)

1. Appendix 1, Source: The list of international conferences has been prepared by the author.

Appendix 2: Health Scheme of the League of Nations for the Establishment of a Permanent International Health Section

1. Rockefeller Archive Centre, RG 1.1, series 100, box 20, folder 165.

Appendix 3: Agreement between the League of Nations Health Organization and the International Health Board of the Rockefeller Foundation

1. Letter from W. Rose to E. Drummond, RAC, RG 1.1, series 100, box 20, folder 165.

INDEX

For Product Safety Concerns and Information please contact our
EU representative GPSR@taylorandfrancis.com Taylor & Francis
Verlag GmbH, Kaufingerstraße 24, 80331 München, Germany